RANT, ...

Chronicl...

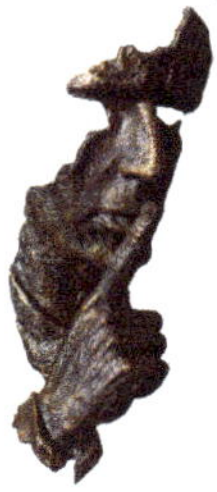

Jimmie Moore

Steel Crow Productions
Jacksonville, Florida

Book Design by Sagaponack Books & Design
Cover Design by Philip Logan
Thanks to Mary Ann Lynn for copy editing and
Frances Keiser for publishing assistance

ISBN 978-1-7326719-3-5 (softcover)
ISBN 978-1-7326719-4-2 (hardcover)
ISBN 978-1-7326719-5-9 (e-book)

LCCN: 2021920183

Summary: The journal of a Vietnam veteran dying from the effects of Agent Orange, and the ranting essays of his friend angered by the military's injustice.

BIO008000 Biography & Autobiography / Military
HIS027070 History / Military / Vietnam War
MED118000 Medical / Military Medicine
MED050000 Medical / Ethics

Steel Crow Productions
Jacksonville, Florida

Printed and bound in the United States of America
First Edition

"This struggle may be a moral one, or it may be a physical one, and it may be both moral and physical, but it must be a struggle. Power concedes nothing without a demand. It never did and it never will. Find out just what any people will quietly submit to and you have found out the exact measure of injustice and wrong, which will be imposed upon them, and these will continue till they are resisted with either words or blows, or with both. The limits of tyrants are prescribed by the endurance of those whom they oppress."

—Frederick Douglas

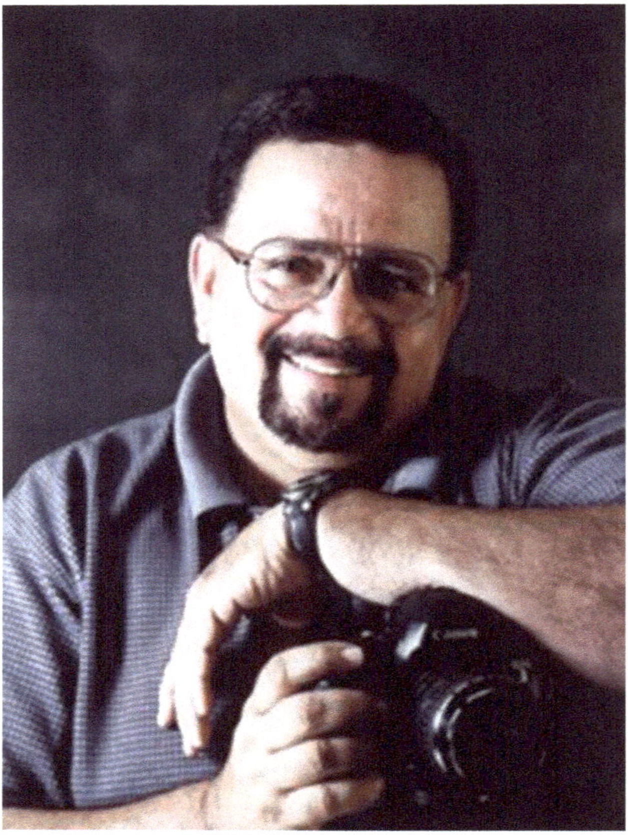

My Friend Joe Barbarisie

He Ain't Heavy, He's my Brother!

DEDICATION

Veterans Administration doctors and administrators are on notice having denied Agent Orange existence, refusing recognition, given no status. Fifty-years creating lies, that ensured the majority of 2,000,000 dead Vietnam Veterans never received any compensation.

Doctors and pharmakia hacks have twisted the VA into a pill palace and slow death. VA hospitals offer only death for the victims of chemical warfare waged in Vietnam. There is no healing, anywhere in the VA infrastructure. Healing is the key word.

Veterans' organizations did not address the Veterans Administration's unwillingness to recognize Agent Orange as the umbrella for all other issues. Never rallying the troops around justice. Never, god forbid, organize the troops for anything. It took fifty-years to kill off 2,000,000 Vietnam Veterans and for the lack of leadership we Veterans failed to resist and make demands.

2,000,000 Vietnam Veterans have given all. Again!!! Most of these 2,000,000 left a bride behind, a family, even grand-babies. The Vietnam Veteran lives the best he knows how. My intentions for *Rant, Whine & Bitch* is to open eyes and then the heart. The whole medical cartel is death, including all VA hospitals. Hiding the data about Agent Orange and chemical exposure, immoral.

Women will one day be called to lead Veteran groups. Their stories are a whole new movement towards justice.

FOREWORD

This is an unusual telling of two stories...

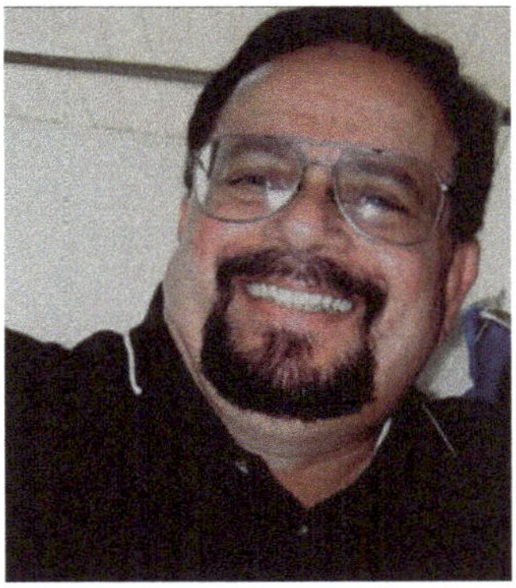

Joe Barbarisie

One is the story of Joe Barbarise, a Vietnam veteran suffering from the later-stage effects of Agent Orange, and mostly written through the journal he kept during the last year of his life in Veteran Administration (VA) hospitals.

The other story is the rants of Jimmie Moore—Joe's fellow comrade in arms and one of Joe's best friends who also has been affected by Agent Orange. Jimmie's rants are selected from his blog at moorek9.com.

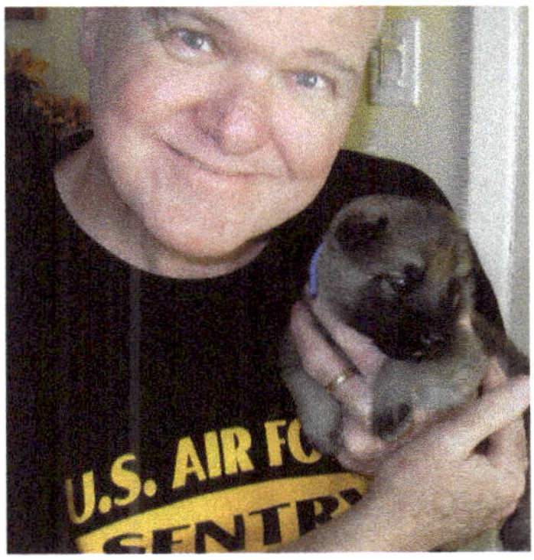

Jimmie Moore

The stories are two very different points of view and written with a different emotional frame of reference. Joe is a gentle man who rarely shows anger and Jimmie is fiery and angry at the injustices that Joe and other veterans and their families faced.

Jimmie is writing this book in the hope that more citizens will become aware of these injustices and help to address them.

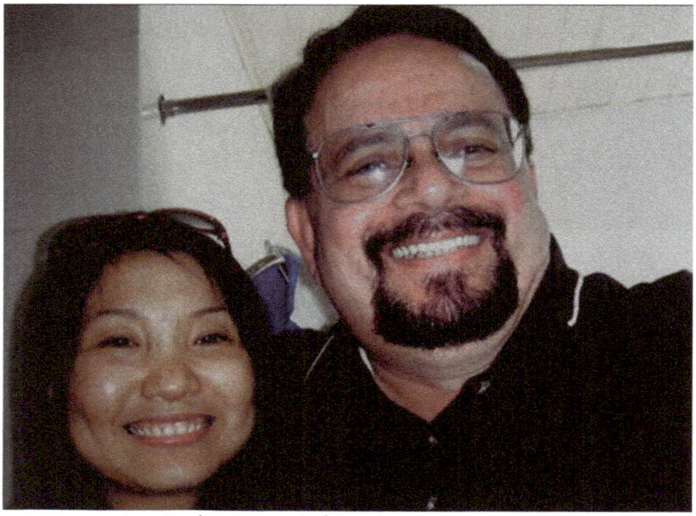

Joe Barbarise with friend, Lee, August 2006

This is when Joe arrived in China. He had taken a position teaching conversational English at a University in Zhengzhou, and also soon became involved teaching and helping orphans and underprivileged children.

I DON'T KNOW WHY

November 24, 2011, Thanksgiving Prayer to Friends

I have been a Christian believing in God my whole life. Sometimes it's difficult. I try to understand why I was chosen to get this horrible, extremely painful, life long illness. I think I'm a pretty good guy. Perfect? Not at all, but reasonably good. I try to help others and teach and lead by example.

While in China I tried to help people as often as I could. It felt like that is what I was made to do. Helping the orphans was the best. In the five years I taught there I had about 1,500 students between all the full-time and part-time jobs I had. I tried to help orphans at three or four different orphanages. I taught my students to be kind, to help others, to donate blood, etc. That's all but over now. Why does God choose to hurt all these people through me?

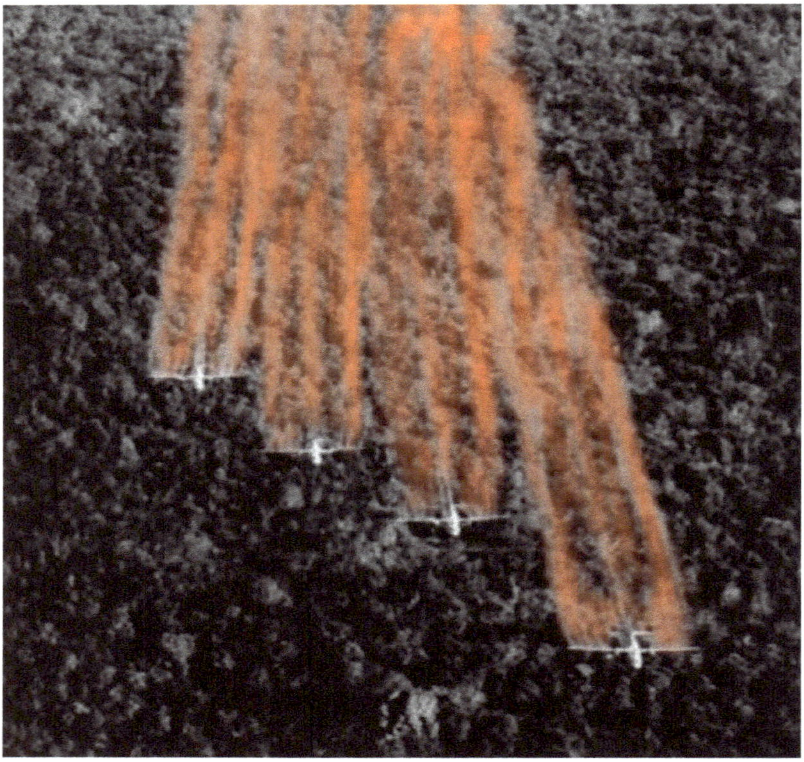

You're looking at chemical warfare, THIS IS WHAT YOUR GOVERNMENT IS CAPABLE OF. The photos in this book, could be YOU next time. This is not a pretty book and is meant for 'on the edge' people who care enough to do something better. Everything about this book is to get people to imagine and create better solutions.

All of my entries and rants in this book have been taken from my blog on MooreK9.com. The thing I like about Blogging is being redundant. The people who care need to be reminded until moved to action.

THE LONG ROAD BEGINS

Joe

December 5, 2009, China

About 4 weeks ago I discovered some small bumps on my head like real bad dandruff and I decided to see a doctor as it looked bad to me. I called Lisa, head nurse at Henan Provincial People's Hospital, and asked her to help. She did. She brought me to the head of Dermatology, Dr. Li. He diagnosed Seborrhea Dermatitis (cradle cap). That is a common condition for babies but rare for adults.

I took medications he prescribed for a week. It got worse. It completely covered my scalp and was now showing on my hair line and neck. I went back to him again. He brought in 3 additional subordinates and they concurred with his diagnosis, maybe because he was their boss. I continued the meds another week, at Dr. Li's recommendation, and I got worse.

A friend from Christmas Coffee named Rose told me of a small, older hospital in Kaifeng that specialized in skin disorders. We went there.

This doctor was much more concerned, gave different meds and strongly advised I go to Zhengzhou University Hospital #1 near my home in Zhengzhou.

I did. It seems I have a rare skin disease called Pemphigus Foliaceus. I never heard of this before and neither has anyone I know. As I dig deeper into the Internet for information, I find it has no cure. I never much thought of those two words before with any ailments I have had in the past. It makes you stop and think.

The lesions spread rapidly completely covering my scalp, continued to my hair line all around my face, my neck, chest, shoulders and back. There is near constant burning and extreme itching. About five years ago there were no medications available for this disease. Treatment and prognosis was easy….get this disease and you die.

A few hospitals world-wide have done very small unreliable studies and developed a treatment. Since few people get this problem, the drug companies do not spend money looking for a cure. Now the doctors use a series of medicines including Prednisone and other similar products, all of which carry severe side effects. Some of the side effects include high blood pressure, diabetes, liver damage, kidney damage, glaucoma and cancer. Remember…these are the "side effects," not the original disease.

I have seen several doctors here and about 6 student doctors. Oh yes, this is a teaching hospital attached to a university. The doctors seemed very nice and concerned. I guess if a foreigner dies while under their care, it's not a high point on their Resume (CV). There are 3-4 different types of Pemphigus with a couple of sub-types to boot. Type one has a strong relationship to prolonged use of any of five different meds. Of course, I never used those meds so that is not mine. By the way, type one is the only one that cures itself by not using those meds any more.

Type two is the one I thought I had, Foliaceus, while my doctor said no, her thought was type three. Only further tests would decide. Type three is over 80% associated with undiagnosed cancer. They administered several tests looking for cancer in the following days.

Two days ago I was told I was cancer free. I could breathe a little more now. The tests continue. They agreed it was type two, Foliaceus, but still need to determine which of two sub-types.

Friends have come to see me. Many friends and students have come. Word has spread across China to my students that graduated last year too. I'm getting calls and text messages from Beijing to Shenzhen wishing me to get well soon.

Many friends bring gifts. Fruit, so much fruit…apples, bananas, many bananas, a case of bottled water, cooked beef, milk, yogurt, fruit juice, big flowers, bigger flowers, small flowers... and my favorite of all...the small gifts bought or personally hand made by my students, all these things designed to bring cheer and happiness to me in my hospital room.

The student union, led by my students, have organized the students to come here in small groups of 2 or 3 to talk with me and act as translators or do anything I need done. It's different here in many ways. Here, if you are in the hospital, you must have another person stay with you. In USA nurses or assistant nurses do everything you need. Not here. Your friend or family member is responsible for your bed, food, bathing, etc.

My best friend here, Will, has arranged for his father to cook and deliver a great Chinese lunch and dinner every day. They bought a special container to transport the food still hot. They live about 30 minutes away and bring the food by bus daily.

Sheralee has stayed here with me every night, all night, after work. She wanted to stay home from work and stay here full-time but I told her no. She must work. She is a mixture of a little bit girlfriend, wife, personal assistant and guardian from all things evil.

During the day, many people, between 1-15 show up to cheer me up. The room is small for the 2 beds that are here. There is a very small seat here for guests to sit on. I had the room to myself for a few days, but that was about to end. They told me I was about to get a roommate. I was not pleased. Like I said it was a small room, but even worse was the fact that if the other bed was taken, then where would Sheralee sleep all night? She would have to sit on that tiny hard seat and lay her head on my bed. I could not have that so I told the nurses that I wanted to pay for both beds in my room. Reluctantly, they agreed. If Sheralee was kind enough to stay here all night, every night, then I had to be sure she was well rested for work the next day.

Every day here is filled with emotions. It's bad enough that I'm not sure exactly what's coming around the corner at me in the next moment, keeping me a bit nervous to say the least, but add to that these unbelievable drugs I must take. One of the side effects is they cause major mood swings. You mean I'm not worried enough? Now these add more to the fire.

The students and my friends have been great. Someone is almost always here to cheer me up. I try my best to be happy, at least on the outside. Sometimes it gets pretty hard to keep wearing a brave face. This disease I have just gave me another shocking moment. One of my doctors came in this morning and told me the sub-type I have of this disease may transform into Lupus. What more can they possible lay on me? I try to keep positive. I try to pray to God to see me through this. I TRY to keep a happy face as the students visit me.

Just a few minutes after I was told about this Lupus bomb, five happy students came to see me. I did not tell them what I was just told. I did my best to conceal the fear inside. Sometimes it swells up so powerful, so consuming, I just lay here and I can feel my heart beating in my chest, so hard it actually shakes my body small amounts. Sometimes my brave face shows signs of wear, maybe a small crack, and a friend sees it. They seldom say so, but I know. They will come closer and hold my hand.

December 22, 2009

It's December 22nd today and I'm still here in the hospital. The days pass quite slowly. Friends and students come to help, but after a while, fewer come. It's natural. They all have school, lives, jobs and families of their own. Two and a half weeks here and I'm healing so slowly.

The problem seems to be the fever they cannot stop. I'm getting IVs every day, the last few days, 10 per day. They switched antibiotics a few times. The days are not well, the afternoons pretty good, then at night the fever returns. About 1-2 hours after I go to sleep it begins. I feel a little cooler at first even though the heater is on in my room. I get a slight tremor in my chest. I try to relax and make it stop. It works a little, but soon worsens and I cannot stop them any longer.

My chest, then my whole body shakes more and more. I call to Sheralee. She brings me hot water bottles to put under the blanket, and then tucks in the blanket well. She adds a second thick blanket, then a third. She then checks my temperature and sees it going up from normal 37° to 38°.

She tells the nurse who now brings the doctor. The staff here is quite concerned about my fever. It's uncommon to not respond to antibiotics. I'm worried too. I should have gone home by now and I will if this fever breaks. Last night there was no fever. I'm quite happy with that. I hope we can do two days in a row with no fever.

My friends in USA, Vince and Jimmie, are the best. Both are trying to find ways to help. Vince with his niece/Doctor and Jimmie with the VA hospital in the Philippines.

The days grew to weeks, four to be exact. Each day I wonder what is in store for me. I read many things on the Internet about this disease....all not good. There was a medicine that was very promising, with no side effects, except for the price. Oh, the price. For a regular size person here, the price was 3000 rmb per day. As the medicine is based on your weight, I needed higher doses, double to be exact. That would be 6000 rmb per day. At an exchange rate of 6.84-1 that's $877 per day, with a five-day cycle needed minimum. That comes to $4,386 per cycle. There may be several or more cycles needed. Highly unaffordable.

Being on the IVs for almost 4 weeks was difficult. I had to sit or lay down 6-11 hours during the day for them to flow properly. These drugs made me need the rest room more, much more. Each time I did, it increased the risk of the IV becoming stopped up with blood reversal. Almost every day it did and they would have to re-do the IV. I had so many holes in my arms and hands that finding a good vein was increasingly difficult daily.

They finally decided to install a long term IV tap that stayed in me for 5-7 days at a time. This made it much easier and less painful to start the IVs but I could not get it wet, so showers were out, sponge baths only, Monday, Wednesday and Friday, the only days hot water was available in my room.

Three days before my fourth week there, they decided to try to wean me off IVs completely and use oral meds instead to get me ready to be released. My body had to be able to handle these new meds and not cause new lesions on my body. They wound up giving me eleven (11) different pills to take between 1-3 times daily. That is in addition to the four insulin shots I need daily also. The pills seem to be working. The doctor warned me that they were sometimes very hard on the stomach as well as other organs and gave me a warning list of things that if any occurred, I was to return to the hospital immediately.

January 3, 2010

It's now January 3rd, 2010 and I have been home [in Zhengzhou] 4 days now. The pills seem to be ok, though quite expensive. The insulin will run 759 rmb monthly. I quote rmb (Chinese money) because I earn rmb here and spend rmb here. Imagine if you will, you spending that amount in dollars. I haven't priced all of them as yet but the blood pressure medicine costs 48.6 rmb for a one-week supply. That's 195 rmb monthly. Blood sugar testing is also expensive. The tabs that read the blood are one-time use. They come 25 to a container, two containers to a box at 270 rmb per box. That equals 162 rmb monthly for those little tabs. I still have many other meds to price.

The hospital stay was about 25,000 rmb plus food. Oh yeah, no food furnished. There is a cafeteria of sorts on another floor where you can order food as you wish but you pay extra. Not good tasting as in most hospitals world-wide, I guess. Friends and students were great. Many students from other foreign teachers came to see me as well. I had bags and bags of bananas, apples and tiny oranges (my favorite), but due to the new found diabetes, fruit was off limits. If I skipped rice for one meal, then I could have one banana.

I have been home a few days now trying to adjust to my new condition and establish some sort of routine. I have been to the drug store several times to stock up on needed items and meds. I can never run out of meds or supplies under any circumstances. I keep examining myself for any new lesions as the doctor asked. None so far but I get ill every time I look in the mirror. I'll admit I was never Prince Charming, but neither was I the latter half of Beauty and the Beast as I appear now.

Two days ago, I spoke with a Chinese lawyer about my illness. I told him how I was misdiagnosed twice from another hospital, delaying my recovery and causing higher doses of meds needed because of that delay, as well as expenses incurred last month as well as future expenses related to pemphigus. He is reviewing some papers during this New Year holiday, but he thinks we may have a case against the other hospital and doctor.

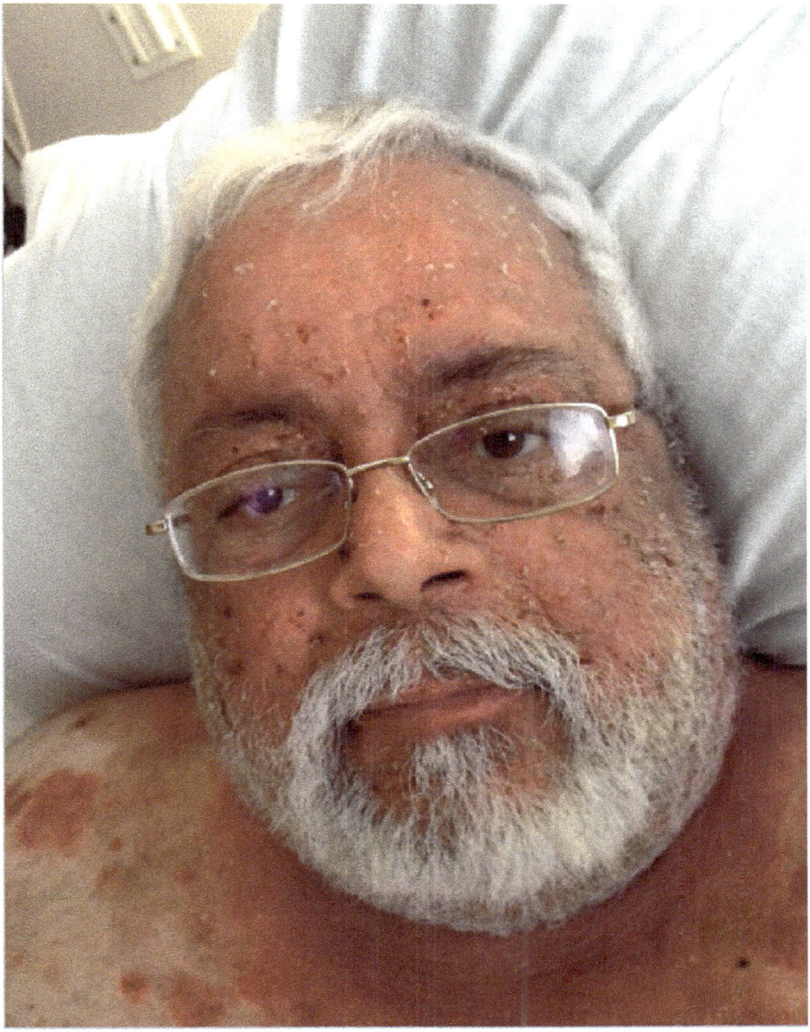

October, 2011. Joe's condition rapidly aged him

I'm Hemp Mellow right now, staring into Joe's sad brown eyes. If you look long enough, you might imagine Joe without the hair on his face. If you freak, that's OK, look into his eyes and feel the warmth, really! Persist. I know what he is thinking here…"Jimmie, I've lost all my dignity!!" I'm glad to visit this picture. It reminds me of a picture of Joe from the neck to belly button that you'll see further along in this book. All these photos should receive a critical eye from you.

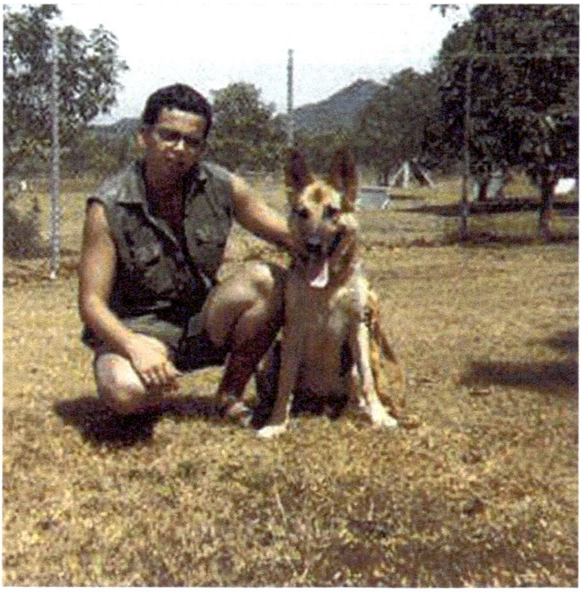

Joseph and Prince, Phu Cat AFB

LIFE'S A BITCH

Jimmie - Rant #1

1968 –

I met Joe in 1968 during Security Police School (SPS), at Lackland AFB. Joe and his hometown friend Vinny befriended me at a time when I was suffering the loss of my girlfriend from a car-train accident back home. Two lives were lost in this tragedy. I was crushed and Joe and Vinny came to my aid and support.

After Vietnam we went our separate ways. Joe to Florida and me to New Jersey. I kept up with Joe through continued contact with Vinny, who was in California. Joe remained in Florida after discharge. He became a Hillsborough County Sheriff Deputy for a time, but his career in Law Enforcement was cut short due to a serious knee injury, incurred while chasing a bad guy down a railroad track. I do not know if Joe was medically retired or not, should have been.

Joe and I were reacquainted after my return to Florida from 20 years of living in Southern California. I spent some time driving Motor Coaches, moving people, and was seeing a lot of Orlando, and dismal-land. Joe was living in Orlando. It was a fun first meeting after so many years. The time Joe was working as a night auditor for several of the large motels in the area. On the surface, Joe was doing okay. He had recently divorced and was living with a roommate when I visited his homestead. The house went up in flames shortly thereafter, with some suspicions in Joe's mind at least and called it foul play. Nothing came of it and he was able to save most of his camera equipment. His big loss were the thousands of negatives of priceless photos of the rich and famous and animalkind.

Joe had a good eye with any camera in his hands. He bought his first camera at the base exchange at Phu Cat AFB, Vietnam. Processed his first negatives on base at a small photo lab set up for airmen to use. He was nineteen years old.

Reunited, we both were a little overweight, in reasonably good health. Joe's crushed knee left him with a slight limp and some pain. Joe lived a comfortable lifestyle in sunny Central Florida, home of Mickey and the gang. But a big change was coming to this laid-back lifestyle in the form of a meet up, with a woman from China who was vacationing in Orlando. This Chinese Women was a college professor and she had an eye out for prospective English teachers and ended up recruiting Joe to come to China and teach Chinese university students English! The change that came over him was priceless. He sold everything he couldn't carry to China in a suitcase and was gone within a matter of weeks. Joe never looked backed. You can still see Joe's blog of his travel log and the first days and months of his arrival in his new home, China, and settling down.

All that needs saying about Joe's Chinese experience is he was happy.

While Joe was enjoying his stay in China, I was several years into my own daily fight to stay alive from the effects of Agent Orange. As I started to slowly regain weight, I felt like I might have a life to live. Joe would be spending a year or so in a Chinese hospital, fighting for his life. Twice he would go into a coma for several days at a time. I communicated with Joe the whole time he spent in China. I knew Joe's health issues were Agent Orange related and begged for him to come home and to get in the VA system, even though I had no faith in the medical care given to Agent Orange victims. I couldn't convince Joe to come home. He had decided to give his last breath, if necessary, to Chinese doctors and medicine. Joe later told me that his doctors were mystified by his condition and deteriorating body. The Chinese medical establishment was getting nervous having never seen anything like the nerves, organs and skin deterioration caused by chemical poisoning. This was totally unknown territory. Luckily, the Chinese government stepped in and ordered Joe home. Joe still did not want to come home.

It was during his hospital stay in China that Joe met the lovely Miss Wangli, one of his nurses.

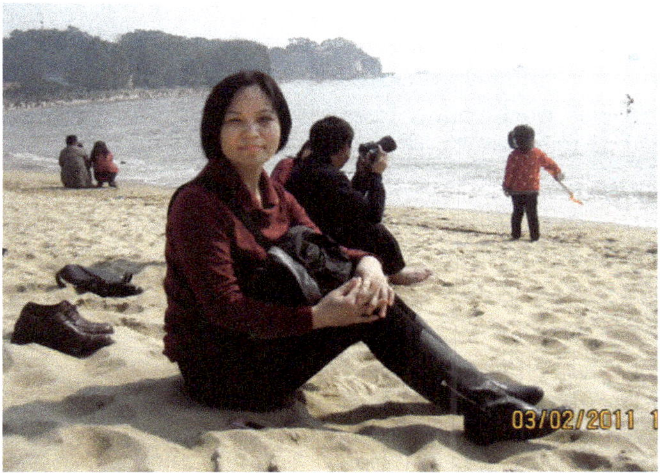

Joe falls hard for Nurse Wangli!

She was married at the time but was in the process of divorcing. They fell hard for each other and had made plans for marriage on his return. I've attempted to get in contact with Nurse Wangli with no luck, my letter was returned unopened. I wonder if my inquiry might have caused problems for her with the Chinese Communist Party. I pray not. I would hate to have that on my conscience. I have not given up on contacting her. All I know about this woman is Joe was madly in love with her. On several of my visits I would get to listen in on their conversations—nothing but puppy love. This woman and the love she gave freely to Joe was key to his many improvements, his zest for life, his desire to live, and his longing to get back to China, get married, and resume teaching. All this love coming from 10,000 miles away from the far east via a smart phone. They talked most days. Joe had someone who cared about him and Miss Wangli was a powerful healing force for Joe.

On his return from China, I met Joseph Barbarise at Tampa International Airport. He was accompanied by two professors from the same University where Joe taught English. Joe looked just awful! He was in a wheelchair, couldn't walk, and was 300 pounds. He had been through a living hell making the trip back to Florida. He told of the difficulty using the toilet while in the air. Joe would not have been able to travel without the aid of the two Chinese professors who accompanied him. A big thank you to those men, they were God sent!

Joe was bed-bound from day one. Just getting his nasty clothes off his body was a task that involved half a dozen or more hospital staff. They had to use a lift to get Joe out of the wheelchair. His screams scared the hell out of me. It took hours of effort and a lot of hard work by staff to get Joe cleaned up and put to bed. Finally, peace came, then sleep and Joe could rest. I got to talk to him the next morning watching him devour his breakfast. What a difference a day makes, and a clean body helps. The trip from China was pure torture, but Joe was home, in a VA hospital and already receiving medicines for pain. His first day back in America was one of tests, followed by countless doctor visits who ordered more tests. I returned to Jacksonville.

After two months Joseph informs me he is being transferred to a rehab hospital in Orlando at the regional VA Hospital. I was furious. I could not believe that moving this sick man was going to do anything good for Joe's health. Joe was making improvements daily. In fact, Joe was doing so well that he picked out a car and bought it, got a new Florida Driver's License. He was barely walking, having to use a walker, but at least he was up and moving on his own two feet. Amazing. Are we going to see a healing? Joe was doing so well that all he talked about was how great China was and how much he missed Nurse Wangli.

With the first of many moves to a different hospital, Joe's life would change forever. This next hospital turns out to be a nursing home for elderly Veterans, all were older than Joe, most used devices to get around. On top of that, the special medications prescribed for Joe did not follow him to Orlando for a week or more. He was still waiting on a special mattress that allowed some comfort for his battered skin condition, but it alsc allowed him to get needed rest. Joe was heavily sedated with several different drugs. The pain he suffered daily was overpowering and disheartening. From my clash with Agent Orange, I knew about the pain he was going through. That one needless move from one VA hospital to another was, in the end, a death blow. Joe never recovers. He was on the VA conveyor belt to a slow painful death. There was no need to move him. Sons-of-bitches@ VA killed Joseph Louis Barbarise. Joe was just a statistic, a clog in the wheel and would be just another number on a growing list of Vietnam Veterans, dead from the chemical warfare of Vietnam colorfully called Agent Orange.

One of the big issues for Joe was his skin sticking to the bedsheets. The doctors had to order a special mattress. I was there a few times when he would try to move, pulling skin loose. I can't begin to describe the pain this caused. Joe had tears in the corners of his eyes most of the time. I was never embarrassed by the different show and tell of Joe's emotions. Pain can make you crazy.

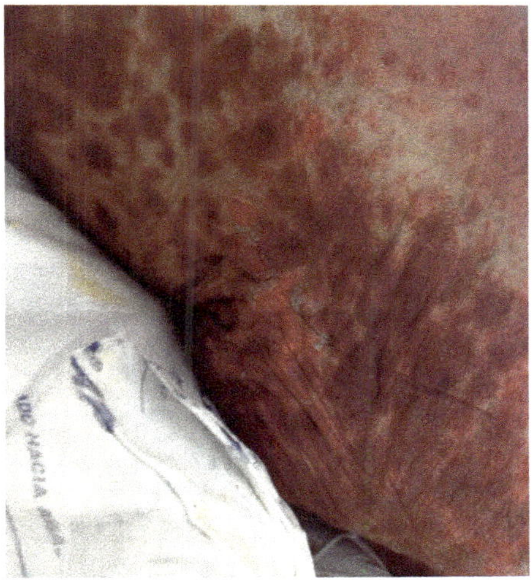

"... he would try to move, pulling skin loose."

"I'm a little nervous. Not sure what's coming." Joe would say this to me several times! But on a positive note, Joe was back in Orlando. Home after all the years absent and he did a lot of re-acquainting with old friends. At first all was well, nice seeing old friends. Then things just stopped happening, like nc baths, lying exposed (naked) for hours, see a nurse at shift change, in and out and gone, forgetting about him and, this the worst of all (the straw that broke the camel's back), wrong soap. I just want you to know, he cried like a baby because staff used the wrong soap. Joe was scared. He faced these demons all alone. He was fighting this thing, this disease that was eating him alive, and it didn't even have a name. This thing, this painful disease was eating Joe alive, body fluids oozed to the surface through the skin. So, The Walking Dead are alive and slowly dying, all over America. We, the walking dead, wait for our number to come up, we fight to live just like back then, (SEA) only to be sacrificed and betrayed again by lying 1%'$, the medical community and the backsliding of the American People for a second time. Isn't America something else.

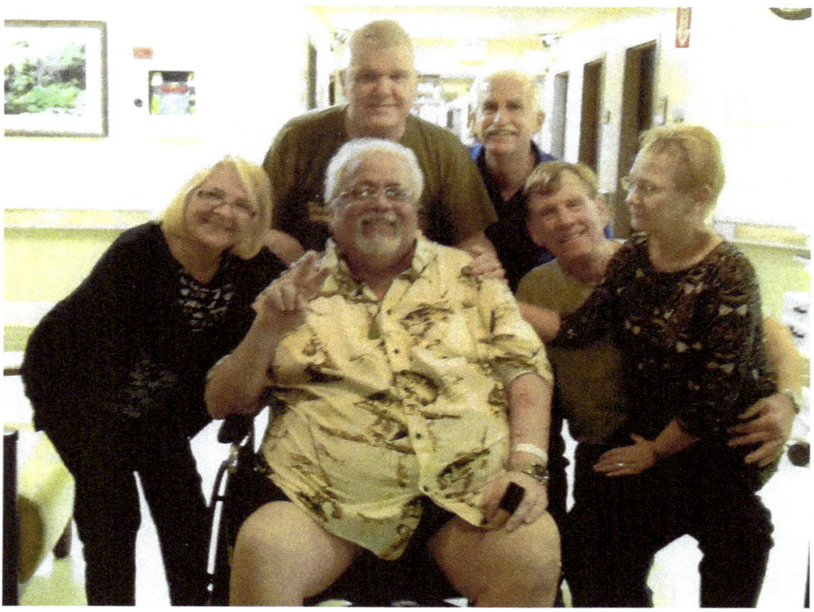

Tell me Joseph Barbarise isn't looking healthy? Damn right he is. As long as doctors' orders are followed, Joe seems to thrive. He secured a Florida driver license and bought a used car. Does that sound like a man preparing to die! Myself and Virginia met up with Vincent and John and Sherry at a Vietnam Dog Handlers Associations (V.D.H.A) meeting being held in Orlando. We traveled the short distance to Tampa VA. We left Joe feeling like he is doing well, he's going to make it. But within a week of this picture, Joe would be moved to a different hospital. My friend never recovered.

VA HOSPITAL, TAMPA AND ORLANDO, FL

Joe

Arrived Tampa VA Hospital, October 8, 2011

Many tests began. October 16th had LP (spinal tap) done. Found protein in spinal fluid. Not good but no reason why yet. Two guys from physical therapy came today. They had me standing a minute or two with lots of help from them. Then they hooked me to an overhead lift system in the room and lifted me into a recliner where I stayed almost three hours. My first time in a chair in about two weeks. I miss Wangli.

Still not all results from spinal. They did a CT scan on October 20. Waiting on those results too. My face is getting a little worse. I'm a little nervous. Not sure what's coming.

Orlando VA Hospital, December 15, 2011

I was transferred to Orlando VA Hospital as I was stabilized and in good shape from Tampa VA. It feels different here. I'm only here a few weeks but everything going downhill here. Sores are becoming visible on my chest, stomach, legs, arms and my back feels strange. I keep telling them something is wrong. I have been here over two weeks and have not even seen Dr. Treat, the one in charge. She has not seen me at all. I mentioned this to one of the nurses and she wrote it in the computer as she must. The next day Dr. Treat saw me in the hall and said hello. Still no physical exam.

January 3, 2012

Approximately (looking back). I spoke to one of the nurses at Orlando VA Hospital about how unhappy I was here. I told her my meds were not given as often as required or not at all. I told her my meds were changed and I was never examined fully by either nurse practitioner Gladys Alphonse or by Dr. Treat, so how can they alter my meds.

My skin condition was much worse due to this treatment. I told her that I did not expect any special treatment but I did expect my meds as required. This nurse wrote this all up in the computer and brought to the supervisor's attention. The next day I was approached twice by Dr. Treat to say hello and see if I was okay. I was also treated and examined by Gladys Alphonse. Now everyone goes out of their way to say hello. I don't want that, just the same treatment as others. A CNA named David came in and said he volunteered to work with me, to help me. About January 11 he was in my room and said he hopes I'm not the type of person that is never happy no matter what others do for him. I was shocked. He was extremely rude with that comment. All I expect is polite staff and all meds in a timely manner.

January 7, 2012

(Approximately) David wrote in computer that I refused my shower that day at 1PM. What he did not say was that I already had a shower at 6AM that day. He also did not mention that I asked him for help with a shower on Saturday, the day before, and he refused my request. Kathy from physical therapy refuses to acknowledge the pain and damage to my skin. She insists that I put on the very tight Jobst stockings alone. I told her several times that my skin under my thighs and buttocks has many open sores, the skin falls off and it is extremely painful. I will be happy to put them on alone as soon as the sores heal. She told nurses and nurse assistants to not help me put them on.

Letter to Senator Marco Rubio, Jan 7 2012

Dear Mr. Rubio;

My name is Joseph Barbarise. I am a resident of Orlando, and a disabled Vietnam veteran. I was forced to return from working in China due to health reasons. On October 8th 2011 I was admitted to James A. Haley VA Hospital in Tampa, Florida. I will try to keep this as brief as possible. About November 2009 I developed a rare auto-immune skin disorder called Pemphigus Foliaceus, possibly from Agent Orange. Twice while in China this went sepsis (blood poisoning) and I was in a coma close to death. Upon arriving in USA, I had lost most motor functions.

At the Tampa V.A. hospital I was treated with respect and courtesy from a highly motivated team of professional doctors, nurses and even clerks who maintained an inventory of necessary medications.

After about eight weeks, on December 12, I was transferred to the Orlando V.A. facility on 5201 Raymond Street Orlando, FL 32803.

This was completely different. Some of the staff are competent, caring people, but several are not. It seems that each nurse or assistant has different ideas as to what I need, even though it's clearly stated in their computers as orders from the doctors. To start, I was on long term Prednisone, being weaned off due to extreme side effects of that drug.. It was being replaced with 1500 mg daily of another drug. It is extremely important that I get the replacement drug daily, as un-medicated outbreaks only take days to flare up, but they take months to get back under control and are quite painful. This facility told me they did not have the drug yet even though they knew I was coming and knew which meds I needed. I told them it was in Tampa and if necessary, I would pay Fed-Ex over night myself. It was three days before I got the drug and my skin is getting much worse.

I have several ointments that I must get twice daily for different areas of my skin. Some I got twice daily, some once and a few times I received none. Some nurses tell me I get an ointment for my face while others say I do not get any. One told me after two weeks the doctor in charge of this unit (Dr. Treat) discontinued that medication for me. I told the nurse I never even saw the doctor at all so how could she change my meds? They said Gladys Alphonse, nurse practitioner (second in command) told her about my condition. Ms. Alphonse has never seen my full condition herself. There was not a complete physical evaluation done even after two weeks. Some nurses tell me I am to get 2 ointments daily, while some tell me 3 and others say 4. There is no consistency. I asked Dr. Treat why this was happening and she told me that she was not able to see my medical records from Tampa V.A. I told her next day I would gladly sign and release if necessary for her to get my records. I could not believe she was not able to see them as she was my doctor and they both worked for the V.A. This time she changed her story and said they were two different computer systems and some of my files were unreadable to her. I asked why she did not order a hard copy to read and she smiled and said nothing. I even brought a complete English copy of my medical records from China so all doctors could be completely up to date on my treatment.

With my disorder its important I practice good hygiene. Ms. Alphonse authorized two showers weekly, not seven as I need. The first week I received zero, none. The second week I received only one. The speaker on my nurse call button has been broken since I got here. I told them three times but it's still broke. I called the nurse on more than one occasion and it took 30-45 minutes for them to respond.

Twice they did not come at all because when they spoke to me on call box I did not answer them. I did not answer because it was still broken. It's still broke. What if I choke or have a heart attack and can't talk and I press nurse call button and no one comes for 45 minutes or not at all? Sir, this is just a sample of what happens here every day. I believe the rules say that all employees be veterans. Many here are not. They are friends of higher ranking veterans. Sir, myself, as well as all other veterans, really need your help. We need a voice that people will listen to. We need you. I come from a patriotic family. My dad served in WWII, my step daughter in the first Gulf War and myself in Vietnam. We are not afraid to serve but hope to get decent medical treatment and respect later in life.

Sincerely,

Joseph Barbarise

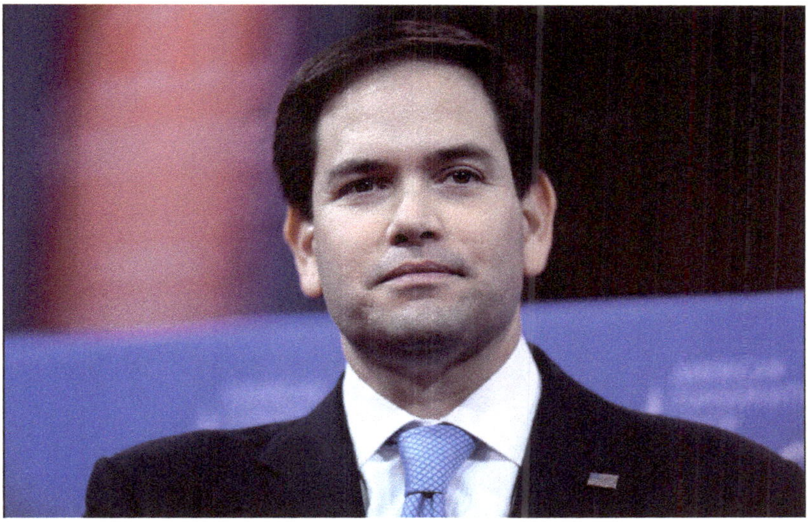

On receiving Joe's letter, Rubio's office in Orlando contacted the head of the Veterans Administration. A staff member informed Joe they were waiting on a reply. Next day a staff member contacted Joe and informed him that the VA was looking into it. Once they moved Joe for the second time, contact was lost with the Senator. No one from Mr. Rubio's office contacted Joe again. Nobody from his office or sent by him, attempted to visit with Joe and see for themselves.

To Joseph, Rubio was a waste of time. Not even a letter came from Mr. Rubio. Again, a Vietnam Veteran is betrayed by another American—this time a senator.

Joe never received compensation from the VA or Social Security, even though in the eight months of Joe's final days he spent a lot of time on the phone with them. I think Joe was ignored intentionally, "just waiting for me to die," Joe would say. Of the two million dead Vietnam Veterans, how many would agree with Joe? I think most!

FALLEN GODS

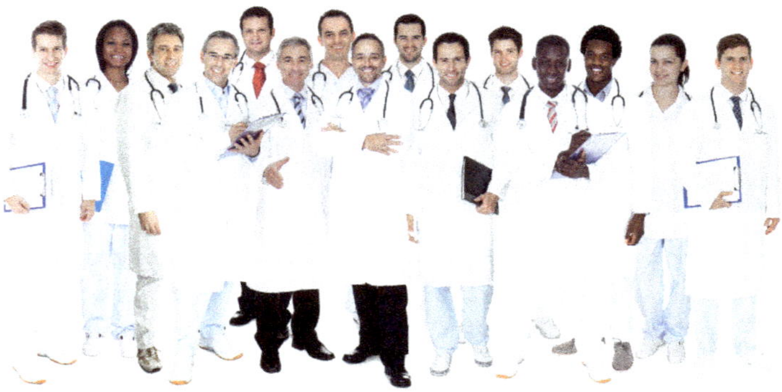

Jimmie - Rant #2

2020

"Tampa is getting ready to ship me out for the second time but not sure where to." Are you kidding me? You talk about stupid is as stupid does!? County after county refused to take Joseph. It took several weeks to finally find a place that would take him, and he ended up in Melbourne, Fla. For those two weeks Joe was informed that he would be moving that day, only to have the move, canceled. Then a new date was set. These other institutions of non-healing could not help Joe. Staff and Doctors had no idea how to deal with chemical poisoning, so they passed. Nobody has ever dealt with chemical warfare and treating the effects of Agent Orange, there was no treatment. There was no instructions guide, no plan for healing. Just a steady stream of pills and services.

They, the VA, did not learn a thing. I was upset the first time they shipped him out. Joe always felt like they wanted his bed, just to make it available to someone else." The sad part was there were few patients in this new wing and there were empty beds. Those first months at Tampa VA were the best two months out of ten months of Joe's hospitalization. Now to move him a second time was criminal negligence. Joe thrived and had a good Thanksgiving.

Then the VA gods made the decision that Joe was stable, had been here long enough and the hospital needed the bed. Joe the Veteran had no say. He didn't want to move; he was happy with the attention to care he was receiving. He liked the staff, everything started right here, from making him feel at home and safe, to medications, physical therapy, doctors from a lot of different specialties and pain relief. His skin looked much better with fewer open sores. Note: Joe had me take pictures just before the move, of his skin and those pictures are proof that Joe was getting better. No open, running scores. A big difference from the first couple of weeks of pure hellish pain that Joe suffered when skin pulled loose, stuck to bedsheets. He was healing.

When Joe was shipped back to Tampa VA he was in bad shape and never again did he get back to that level of healing of the first two months, and truthfully, I'm not sure if there was any improvement in Joe's health, not how he felt, but overall health. When I found out about the second move, I was angry and feeling hopeless not being able to help Joe who was freaking out. He was scared. I wanted to scream. Not being a relative I was voiceless. Joe had to make all the important decisions, sign all the paperwork, and try to understand what was happening. Joe did not have an advocate, nobody to secure his right to life. He was alone and naked and getting worse instead of better. Joe was scared. In my heart I felt this move was not going to improve his health, only worsened it. As you read Joe's story you will see how thoughtlessly cruel these moves were. In the end, it ensured his premature death. The Dragon Brigade welcomes Joseph Barbarise.

VA HOSPITALS, ORLANDO AND TAMPA, FL

Joe

January 9, 2012

Approximately (looking back) at Orlando VA Hospital. Nurse Manager Ms. Hernandez came into my room with about eight other nurses, CNA's, etc. and asked to hear my story about missing meds. I told them and she promised me they would never run out of meds again.

She had all others leave and she stayed awhile with me. She asked me my opinion of the problem. I told her she had two problems, one was ignorance and the other was stupidity. The ignorance was easy to solve with a little additional training. The stupidity was much more difficult as those people did not know they were stupid and would not improve with training as they thought they were doing well now. She agreed.

January 15, 2012

Yesterday evening, I was due for my meds on my skin. They ran out AGAIN, even after I was promised it would never happen again. Ms. Chen called the pharmacy on call and told them my medicine was needed. They refused to bring it. They promised they would bring it before 9am Jan. 16. They lied again. It arrived at 11am. That was another 14+ hours with no medication on my skin.

January 19, 2012

At 3:50 PM I requested a nurse help me with a bandage falling off my right upper arm and it was very painful. I used the call button and was told the nurse would be notified and would be here soon. One hour later I called again as no nurse ever responded. I was told the nurses just started. That's a lie. Afternoon shift starts at 3:30 in report room and handles patients at 4:00 pm. Day shift handles patients until 4:00. At 4:10 a nurse assistant came to take vitals. Still no nurse has showed up. Both upper arm bandages have fallen off now. At 5:50 PM, still no one came. Dr. O (psychiatrist) came to see me about 2 PM today. We talked a bit about depression. I told him about my strange family relationship, my house burning down, my poor health and the great deal of pain I was experiencing. I told him Dr. Treat was supposed to give me something for pain this morning but as of 2 PM I still have not seen her. Dr. O said he would go get her and come "right back." It's now 6 PM and he too has not returned. It seems most people here have a very hard time following through with promises. I have to wear compression devices on my lower legs whenever I'm up to control swelling.

January 20, 2012

(Yesterday) I tried to get someone from 2 PM to 8 PM to help me put them on with negative results. This morning I tried from 8am to almost 2 PM before someone came to help. I am diabetic and must have meals and insulin on a regular schedule. Lunch is usually served at 12:15 PM. When there was no meal at 1:15 PM I pressed the nurse call button and asked if there was a meal for me. I was told, "Sorry but we forgot about you". Five minutes later the meal arrived. The insulin arrived another hour later. It should be injected ten minutes before the meal or at the same time.

January 20, 2012

Today, they decided to change my room from #128 to #130 at about 2:00 PM. It is now 8:00 PM and they are still not finished even though the rooms are only two rooms apart.

January 21, 2012

Friday. I got a call from Congressman Rubio's office. They got my letter and called the leader of the V.A. in Washington D.C. to let him know what was happening. I believe he called the Orlando V.A. Hospital Monday morning. Monday morning Dr. Treat, Gladys Alphonse and Ms. Hernandez all came to my room asking how I was and what they can do for me. I don't want special treatment, I just want my meds and treatments on time as ordered. I want to heal and leave soon as possible.

January 25, 2012

We all decided I was in such poor shape I should be transferred back to Tampa V.A. Hospital. I was taken there by ambulance that afternoon and brought into the E.R. for examination. Several staff there remembered me from last time I was there, including one doctor from dermatology. He has four names and the first one is Jean. He was shocked at how poor I looked compared to when I left. I was admitted to the hospital.

The first day here I was seen by at least four different teams of doctors, including but not limited to, dermatology and internal medicine with two to four doctors in each group. Each showed a sincere concern and at least 5-6 doctors visit/examine me. They even had a bone density scan done to me due to the extreme time and high dosage of 120mg daily of prednisone prescribed by Orlando. Tampa had me weaned to 5mg daily before my transfer. It takes a long time to be weaned. Continued usage attacks heart, lungs, liver, eyes, bones and more. Sudden removal can cause death.

The doctors and nurses here in Tampa V.A. Hospital are fantastic. If you look into their eyes, you can see they really care for the patients. I mean really care. In Orlando it's different. Some care but most [they only] act like they care.

Tampa is getting ready to ship me out for the second time but not sure where to. Social Services has struck out in Orlando, Orange County, Hillsborough County and they are now trying to find a bed in Melbourne and Leesburg. The doctors here in Tampa had to lance an infection on the back of my neck

February 8, 2012

They may have to do another on my right cheek as its very swollen and infected too. Dr. Johansen came by today and brought me a coffee. She is so sweet.

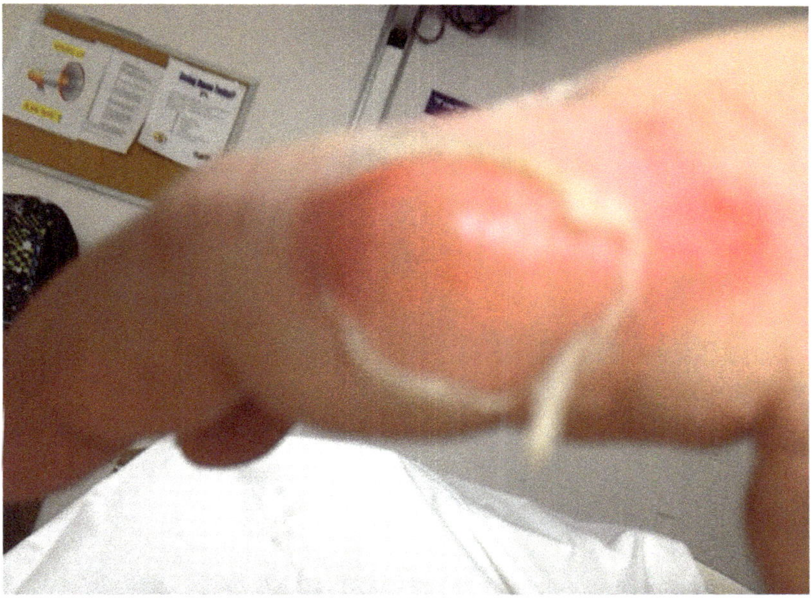

"Now, day by day I can feel my body slipping away, getting weaker."

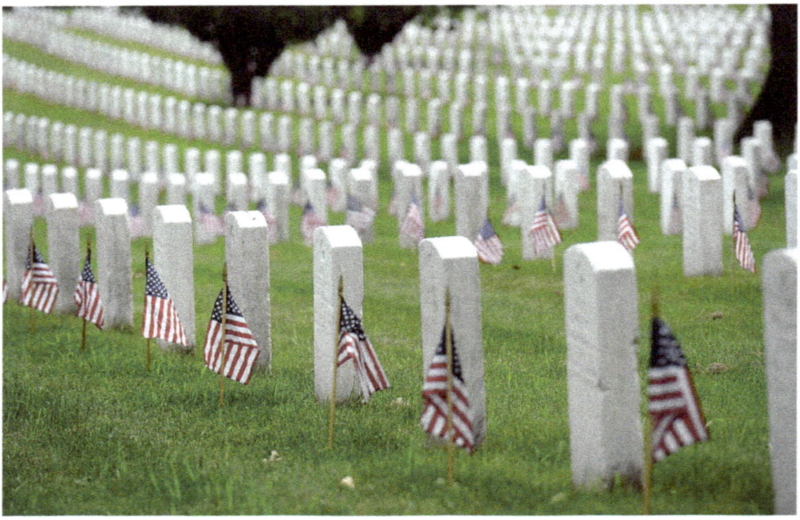

"If only I could put 2 million gravestones from end to end and see where I would end up."

Jimmie - Rant # 3

Did you see how quickly they had Joe shipped to his second medical hospital from N. Melbourne. They were asking Joe to sign away what few rights he had left, mainly the God given abi ity to heal, backed-up with the promise from Uncle Sam to care for the wounded. Now on the other hand, I'm a 100% disabled Vietnam Veteran, I receive a fare pension and with Social Security, me and wife do OK, living below the poverty level.

Every time Joe was moved it was by ambulance, with him on a stretcher and a bedsheet to cover his nakedness. A lot of things had to come together when Joe moved; medical records of medications and treatments prescribed by doctors. Special mattress, taking days or weeks to arrive, etc. Luggage that made it home from China, was now scattered between Tampa, Orlando, Melbourne 1 & 2. Joe still has four more moves and four months of tortured suffering before making the last move, the shortest one to V.A Hospice. Joe arrived to Hospice naked, covered with a bed sheet. He left this world the same way.

July 2, 2019

Two Million Vietnam Veterans are dead from Agent Orange exposure. If only I could put 2 million gravestones from end to end and see where I would end up. Or see how many football fields it takes to plant all the markers. Why is it when it comes to counting the real cost of this war, the 'Walking Dead', the real 'Walking Dead' are ignored? Why are words like murder, genocide, holocaust, and Justice not talked about? There is a big black-hole and Vietnam Veterans are disappearing off the face of the planet.

So, Joe and I conceived the idea of doing an expose' about what Agent Orange does to the body. As Joe's condition quickly got worse, he became like the 'Walking Dead'. From the moment Joe arrived at the Tampa V.A. Hospital until he died in V.A. hospice care in Gainesville, he never wore clothing again. When he was transported from Tampa V.A. to Orlando V.A. nursing home, then back to Tampa, then from Tampa V.A. to another retirement home in Melbourne, FL, from there to a local medical center in Melbourne, from there Joe was transported to Daytona Beach but never arrived, finally ending up at Shand's Teaching Hospital on the campus of the University of Florida, from there, he is moved to a local rehab/nursing home, and finally his last move was to the V.A. Hospital in Gainesville. All this time, the miles in the back of ambulances, Joe was covered in a bedsheet, same as in a bed in a room. Naked and alone!

I visited Joe all over the State of Florida, most weeks, wherever Joe was sent off to, I visited.

Thinking Out Loud

This book is starting off feeling strange. It's not the subject matter, I was a witness. I took the pictures, encouraged Joe to keep a record of day-to-day events, which is Joe's Journal. The V.A. doesn't allow 'easy' access to the internet. Joe got creative and invested in a top-of-the-line iPhone. With it, he was able to stay in touch, but more importantly, he started a log of events for each day. Every few days, messages came from Joe, and I created a file. He understood the need for documenting, as much as possible, his day-to-day life. Joe spent a lot of time texting, documenting his health care and all sent by iPhone. I guess the problem I'm having is me having to write this story at all. Where are the great minds? Where are the 'watchmen'? Why this duty is fallen to a dog handler to tell Joe's story is the crushing reality of a nation that does not care. Why is genocide being put on the backs of the Servicemen who served in

Vietnam? Just disappear, go away, there is no grateful nation. Nobody knows about Agent Orange thanks to media blackout, medical lies and denial, congressional no-interest. A President who refuses Medical Hemp for Veterans. A President who does not declare a national emergency with 22 Veterans committing suicide a day. The Warrior is expendable, is the message being sent and received. The Military Industrial Complex is pathetic. Fear Robots.

But hear this, Joe and I decided to do something about it! So, we planned the book out. Joe was a big fan of my 'the big screen vision' of "Noble Canine" the movie. He would have written the script, had he lived. I jumped at Joe's idea for making "Noble Canine" available in China. Joe had a special relationship with his University Students who were learning English. He feared disappearing, without a trace, that his beloved students would forget him. "Noble Canine" would give a focus and a home, so at least his students would know that going home to America did not save him. The only thing Joe insisted on was the price "Noble Canine" would sell for to students. He liked the sound of .99 cents a copy. I readily agreed. You kidding me, me selling my book in China, to the children of his students, me selling books or anything in China. Having something worthy to read by English students in China, I was blown away by the possibilities. Joe said on a visit one day, he hoped to live and see the day the book is published.

July 3, 2019

I was grateful to the two gentlemen-professors who escorted Joe from China, thru Chicago and finally, Tampa Bay. I think they got the first available flight back to China. The Chinese Government honored Joe, and they did not abandon him in his hour of need. For a year Joe was a guest in a Chinese Hospital, (I think Joe had to pay the hospital bills as he went) their Doctors didn't know what they were dealing with and the government had no choice but to put Joe on a flight back to the world. I had sent several emails urging Joe to return to the States, but he decided to stay and put his fate in Chinese medicine. I was fit to be tied. I knew what Joe was going thru and I had beaten the beast in my own battles with Agent Orange, sort of. My thinking was to get Joe back in the States and under V.A. care and maybe Joe could turn his ordeal around. I had no idea how bad of shape Joe was in until I met him at the airport. It was a short distance to the V.A. Hospital and a big relief for everyone to have Joe safely delivered. I had stopped by this V.A. earlier, before meeting Joe's plane and informed the Emergency Room staff on duty that a Vietnam Veteran was being picked up at the Airport and will be delivered in a couple hours.

Once Joe was brought into an examining room, the staff immediately set to work, getting Joe out of soiled clothing, and filling out paperwork. To get a 300-pound Joe out of his dirty pants required lifting him out of his wheelchair, using straps underneath him and this was killing Joe. He let out a blood-curdling scream and I knew Joe was in some serious pain, with life-threatening issues. It was slow, slow progress, but with a lot of patience from a dedicated staff and about two hours of hard difficult work, Joe was finally in his birthday suit and feeling better about the end of his long trip. All he wanted to do was sleep. I caught a glimpse of Joe as the staff got Joe cleaned up and ready for bed. When our eyes met, I gave Joe a thumbs-up, all Joe could do was shake his head up and down as a response. The body I saw that day and I would see again, even taking pictures, was not a body at all. He looked like someone had poured acid on his body from head to toe. Total shock, total disbelief at what I was looking at. Is this going to be me in my on-going battle with Agent Orange. OMG Help me, Help Joe! I was in tears of disbelief, and I hurt for my friend.

July 4th 2019

I will deviate for a moment and tell you about my visit to a local chapter meeting of the VVA. My first meeting of 2019. One of the speakers was from an organization known as 'Concerned Veterans for America Foundation' and two representatives who were both veterans, spoke on the new effort by the VA, called, VA MISSION Act.

Sorry, just more fluff for us dummies to try and sort-out. The VA is a ghost town when it comes to leadership. Don't confuse VA with HEALING, oxymoron, to say the least.

The VVA served great BBQ to about 20 or so souls. Got informed about the AGENT ORANGE TOWN HALL meeting in August, I had already signed up for this meeting. Then I was informed about a BREAKFAST WITH OUR HEROES, at Applebee's also in August.

During this meeting of Vietnam Veterans, nothing was said about Agent Orange during the Mission Act talk, I was handed a leaflet about the Town Hall meeting, a small mention about Agent Orange during this meeting. Finally, heard the bad news of another recent death and another Vietnam Veteran was in the hospital, and not expected to live.

Dying like flies! The Walking Dead! Not much on conversation when it comes to Agent Orange. Another funeral, another color guard, 21-gun salute, and taps and go home, take your meds, and wait your turn to die. By all means suffer in silence and shut up. Sarcasm.

At this meeting I saw something else, scarier, the 'Walking Dead', knew they were dead fish. You could see it in their eyes. Empty Betrayal. Presumptuous Death, the VA would call it!

It's been six months since I attended a meeting, and this meeting was 50% smaller. This time there was no color guard. To many have died. The last thought of the night concerned what's to become of the VIETNAM VETERANS of AMERICA organization/brand when there are not enough veterans to have a meeting.

My thoughts: If you change the name of the organization, then the Vietnam War will disappear from history is assured. Same as Pearl Harbor is slowly disappearing from history.

How could we allow the murderers of 2 million Vietnam Veterans to get away with this GENOCIDE? This is murder!!

I made a small contribution to the meeting by announcing my intention to interview surviving spouses of Agent Orange victims. I want to hear from the Brides of Vietnam Veterans. I know what they have lived through!

July 1st was our 47th wedding anniversary. The last ten years of our lives together has been taken over by Agent Orange and surviving. Thankful, Virginia!!

I am glad I attended this VVA meeting. Good People, Good Food. But, I must say, the life force is being sucked out of the organization.

Something else is bothering me. I feel a sadness coming over me as I realize our days are numbered and shortened. But I am far too mad to sit still, be still and 'shut up'! Not going to happen! Vietnam Veterans will stand!

A Call to Action:

What the chemical cartel as well as the oil cartel have done over the last 100 years is to systemically destroy the Earth's ability to provide habitats for its creation. AnimalKind is starving and leaving their wilderness homes and ending up in villages, towns, and cities all over the world, eating our garbage. With GMO's invading our food supply, natural farming will die, if not stopped. Earth is threatened. Our home is threatened.

I feel it is our duty as Veterans and as victims of mass chemical poisoning to stop oil and chemical poisoning or this planet will die.

Sooner or later we victims of Agent Orange are going to have to face the fact that leadership in Veterans Organizations betrayed Vietnam Veterans to the ravages, the suffering, the horror of death by the government created Agent Orange. We are sick and old, not dead! There is much that we can do, there is nobody else. We must accept responsibility for the survival of planet Earth. Two generations or 50 years, time is short. Must act.

As I compile this foundation for a book, I will be talking about different events as they come up. Today I went to a town hall meeting about Agent Orange, held at the University of North Florida in Jacksonville. A good turnout, maybe a few heads over 300 people attended. I knew better than hope for LEADERSHIP to finally make an appearance at a Veterans Club Meeting. It didn't.

Same ole Gate-Keeper bull shit. Always talking about the wrong things. Always misdirecting. You Men who have called yourselves Presidents and Commanders of veterans groups, what are you going to do when the remainder of living Vietnam Veterans, their wives, their children, all who fight every day to live, these the survivors of mass genocide by chemical poisoning, created by government-corporate collusion, how will you react when "WE" fully understand the depth of the betrayal to VET GROUPS by those in Leadership. Damn the gatekeepers!

Leadership failed its membership by taking the lights off Agent Orange and sweeping it under the rug. We Veterans, not hearing the truth about the seriousness of the poisoning, ending up doing the dirty work for the chemical companies and the government. I firmly believe if Vietnam Veterans had known the truth about Agent Orange, there would have been a totally different outcome. As it was, the Chemical cartel was given a blank check to proceed with creating GMO's. "Better Living Through Chemistry" is death to the planet. Veterans have no choice but to get involved and bring the global chemical and oil cartels to their knees. As few as our numbers have become, we are the only ones who can stop this worldwide madness, stop this worldwide greed, stop the killing of Planet Earth!

While Joe was in the hospital, the only visitor received was a visit from D.A.V. and I called them and asked them to visit Joe. I called them once in Tampa and again in Orlando. No VVA showed up, no VFW showed. Nobody took any interest in Joe for any reason. Joe basically died alone.

That's the typical story of a typical Vietnam Veteran's experience, dying from Agent Orange. Joe wasn't married, so no immediate family. So, he literally died naked and alone. Married Veterans were lucky because of the safety net provided by our incredible Wives. Veterans could be cruel to wives, who were the only support a man being ravaged by chemical poisoning had. Example: twenty, thirty years ago you didn't see wives attending reunions the way they have to attend these days with husbands so sick they can hardly walk. My wife is why I am alive today and yes, I was mean and hateful and ungrateful. A real jerk. My wife saved me again when she put it together that all the medication

I was on was messing with my mind in a very negative way. I was taking so much medication for pain I was slowly but surely closing organs down. That was going to kill me as quickly as the Agent Orange that ravished my body. A year ago, I made a major decision and resumed smoking cannabis. I dumped the VA meds regime and replaced it with Medical Hemp and smoking the weed. Started feeling better, my aggressiveness went away, peace returned to my home. I would not change a thing except the price. Veterans should not have pay out of pocket for medical hemp or smoking hemp. More betrayal of Vietnam Veterans by government, the AMA, the VA and the President of the United States government and our Commander in Chief of the military who have turned their backs on sensible health care, that still allows for a Vietnam Veteran to be arrested for pot use. Sick. This must stop. It is genocide! Written this day of August 7, 2019.

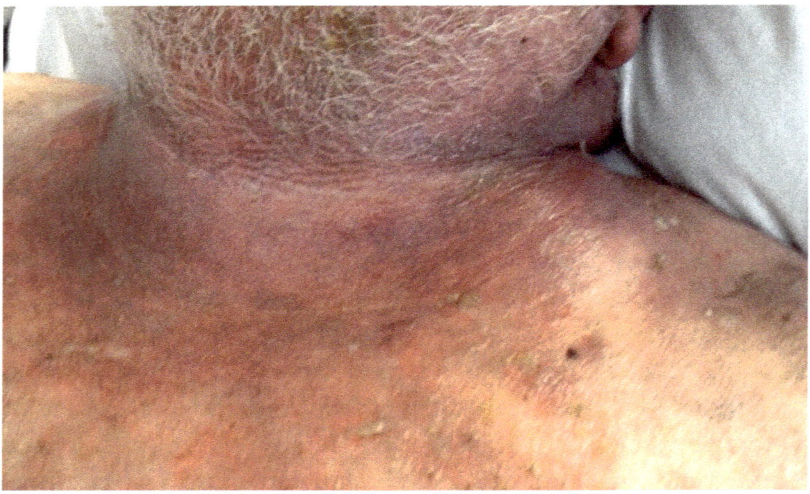

"I was due for my meds on my skin. They ran out AGAIN, even after I was promised it would never happen again."

MELBOURNE, FL

Joe

February 15, 2012

Dr. Poetter faxed my med list to the facility in W. Melbourne (where I would be transferred to against my choice on Feb. 16) to be sure they would have all my meds on-hand including the special air mattress for my skin condition.

February 16, 2012

Upon arrival my heart dropped to the floor. It was exactly as I expected........an "elephant's graveyard" where people are warehoused with minimal care until they die. The ones I've seen are 70-90 years old, many handicapped. This place is a converted old motel, very little converted.

My first day here they had none of my meds on-hand, no IVs, pills, creams, nothing. They said my room was not ready until tomorrow so they put me in this dilapidated room overnight and said I would be changed in the morning.

February 17, 2012

It's now 10 AM and I'm still in an unpainted, unfinished room with things ripped off the walls. My meds arrived 5am today.

I told them last night I needed an elevated toilet seat as getting up from a standard seat was impossible. The seat never came last night or so far today. I was told to call the nurse when I needed to go and she would be sure I could make it ok. I called this morning.

No one came. I reached the toilet but could not stand afterwards. I pulled the nurse call button again from the toilet. It took another 15 minutes to get help to stand. After getting in bed the nurse left without even offering a sheet to cover my naked body.

When I left Tampa, I was told my things would not fit in the ambulance, only about half would. Now they say they will ship my things if I pay. Okay, I'll pay but I have almost nothing here. I asked nurses here three times to please look through my things and see if I have any clothes here I can wear. No one has looked yet. 10:30am the raised toilet seat arrived.

Late this afternoon several staff members came to visit, including the RN, activity lady, a doctor and admitting lady. The RN welcomed me to their facility cordially as did activity lady. The admitting lady had me sign many papers to be admitted including Living Will and DNR. One paper she asked me to sign was a binding arbitration form stating I can never sue anyone there no matter what happened. I refused that one. Less than an hour later I was told I'm leaving this facility, they were transferring me to a local hospital here in Melbourne and would not return here again.

An ambulance arrived and took me to the hospital where I was admitted and placed in ICU. After a three-minute exam that he feared I had or would develop DVT or deep vein thrombosis and then quickly go septic. There were no signs of either, other than the same edema I've had for some time. The hospital ran an ultrasound on my legs to look for clots. Still waiting on results at 12am.

February 17, 2012

8am....test results from DVT test negative. No blood clots at all. Still in ICU but may get moved to regular room today. The staff here at this hospital is excellent. I may be here for the duration of my IVs about one week. After that, I don't know.

February 19, 2012

It's Sunday. My skin continues to improve. I'm getting IVs and other meds as scheduled. Nurses here continue to be very kind. I'm still in ICU area. Jimmie called. He and Virginia will visit tomorrow between 11-12.

February 20, 2012

Jimmie and Virginia arrived at 10:30 AM today. What a great feeling to see them. They stayed until 1pm before starting their long ride home. Two hours after they left the staff here moved me to a regular room still on third floor. It's a beautiful, clean, private room but the mattress is uncomfortable on my skin. They said I might get the air mattress tomorrow. The nurses made me as comfortable as possible. The wound care nurse looked me over and took pictures of my skin.

February 21, 2012

The special air mattress arrived today.

February 22, 2012

Three gentlemen from local D.A.V. came to see me this morning, a pastor and two officers. They contacted the social worker in this hospital and we talked. The social worker will talk to others here about either me staying here awhile to recover, or move me to a rehab she knows locally and move me there. She will make some calls and let me know.

The physical therapy woman came yesterday and we talked and I exercised with her awhile. I also got up and walked with her. Very nice lady. She will come back about three times a week.

WHY COULDN'T HE HAVE LANDED IN ORLANDO?

Jimmie Rant - # 4

Same ole shit. People in 'The system' have come to hate Joseph Barbarise!!! Hate runs to fear and 'The System' had bit off a mouthful of 'dying from the inside out'. The real 'Walking Dead' has come home to roost.

These so-called 'doctors' didn't know how to solve the problem that Joseph Barbarise dropped on their front doorsteps. "Why couldn't he have landed in Orlando"? The 'doctors' had quickly run out of 'any kind of facility' willing to take him in. Imagine what Joe was feeling, his body and mind are racked with pain, and enough medication to kill a horse just to keep him calm and barely able to focus. Forcing Joe out of Tampa VA Hospital for a second time, criminal negligence. Try and imagine Joe's panic and fears! Each new day you're being shipped out, not knowing where, and the VA can't locate a hospital willing to take on Joseph Barbarise and all his many plagues? Tampa VA's list of refusals were counted by counties. From Tampa to Orlando to Daytona Beach is a high-density corridor with many medical accommodations with various specialties and services. It took two weeks of rejection to finally come up with a nursing home in North Melbourne, Fla. With this move, 'The System' signed, sealed, and delivered the next pre-mature death of Joseph Barbarise. The Dragon Brigade numbers are Legions.

Joe managed to document all thirty pages worth of notes about his care as a VA System/patient on an iPhone. Tiny iPhone. Sick, with incredible pain and the medication to deal with the pain, all of it left Joe weak, confused and exhausted. I impress upon the reader the strength of Joe's will.

IVIG, when doctors first introduced this IV to Joe as a new drug and it would become part of doctors approved treatment plan, and the only treatment plan that Joe received during his 8 months VA care, the IVIG was sold as a possible miracle drug. Joe was excited about this new drug and put much faith and hope in it as the first IV was administered. Joe began to feel better but was still dealing with a lot of issues. Joe had good days and bad days, but the one constant was the pain. Agent Orange is illegal under international law. The United States thinks in can get away with murder. Joe commented to me one day the pain felt like fire-ants were eating the very nerve endings, then pissing on raw nerves. The pain Joe suffered was meaner than my fire ants, more liken to a fire breathing dragon. See photos!

The price tag placed on two bottles of this IVIG was $10,000. It took ten hours of slow drip to administer. Joe said it made him feel better. But as time went on, Joe did not get better. Joe had two months of living left. Surviving these last two months was all about enduring pain. Nobody would take responsibility for a dying Joseph Barbarise. Joe was moved 9 times in eight months. Never should have moved him! Never, not even once! Agent Orange is a killer and Joe was walking dead even as he disembarked at Tampa International Airport.

If you have faith in God, faith in America, faith in a doctor, then you should be able to have faith in hope. When the light goes out of your hope then the spirit dies. The will to live can't compete with chemical warfare, the body has no defense.

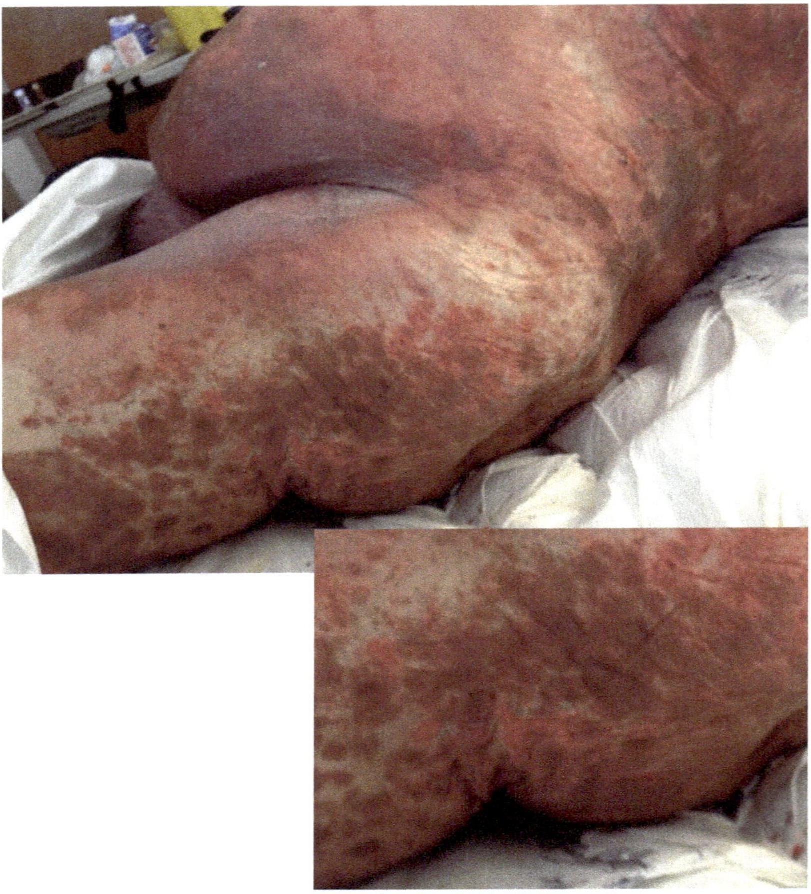

Taking these pictures was upsetting. Try and imagine the intense pain suffered by 2,000,000 Vietnam Veterans who died before their time.

This open wound (enlarged, lower right) was caused by skin sticking to the bed sheets. The problem was greatly improved with the use of a special mattress used for burn victims. A steady flow of air helps to separate skin from sheets. It keeps the skin cool and dry. Without the mattress, Joe could not rest. Without the mattress, every time Joe moved, skin would stick to the bed sheet. Very painful coming off. The VA knew how important using the mattress was, but every time Joe was moved to a different hospital, it took a week or days for the mattress to make its appearance. Same was true for medications. This is insane. Just another example in a long list of poor medical care provided by doctors and nurses at a VA Hospital.

MELBOURNE, FL

Joe

February 28, 2012

Last 7 days my blood sugar levels have crashed four times; twice, dangerously low. Anything under 70 is cause for immediate concern. Mine has run 65, 59, 44 and 39. The 44 and 39 scared me. I was seeing blue spots in front of my eyes and could not respond well to others. I was very weak and dizzy. Two cups of orange juice did nothing. They had to give me pure sugar to eat and still had to give me sugar I.V. I'm getting concerned that response to the nurse call button is extremely slow, 10-30 minutes, or not at all. I told one of the doctors but it was no help.

March 1, 2012

One of the nurses came into my room today and said; oh, it's good to see you. How is your heart? No more heart attacks? Is your heart feeling better? I was worried you might not make it.

I thought, oh my god, I have a bad heart, I'm dying and no one told me. What else are they hiding from me? I was so scared I was white. The nurse looked at me again and said: oh, I'm so sorry but I thought you were Mr. Smith.

March 3, 2012

My feet and legs feel strange today. They are getting bigger. They are swelling very much. I told the nurse and she made a note in my file. My feet actually hurt they are so big.

March 4, 2012

One of the doctors came by today to see my feet. With his accent he is hard to understand. He said he was aware of the swelling and knew why. He said he could control it with no problem. He said something about sulfa but I'm not sure what. Tomorrow is Monday. I'll wait and see what he does then. The open sore on the back of my left calf is pretty bad. It's been there for a while now and got worse today. I had to get up to use the toilet and when I did, I did not notice how badly the skin ripped off that spot. It bled for a few minutes, running down my foot and onto the floor. I called the nurse and showed it to her.

March 6, 2012

At 11AM a doctor just came in to see me. I showed him two new outbreaks on my skin on my sides, both left and right. I don't think that's what he was looking to hear. He kept saying we need to transfer you to rehab, but I don't think anyone will take you. He asked me, "what can we do?" He said I need to be at the V.A. facility. I agreed. He asked several times why Tampa rehab transferred me. I said you have to ask them. I believe they might be a short term at Rehab D, and a very long waiting list for the other areas of rehab.

Oh, I almost forgot. At 11pm last night they decided to move me to another room, another floor. It took until about 1 AM but I was moved to room 2411.

March 9, 2012

I was supposed to start my IVIG this morning and again tomorrow morning. The doctor here was extremely slow researching my file to find out about this. The IVIG is very slow. It takes 8-10 hours to complete. They finally ascertained that I was supposed to get it and started the IV at 7 PM. He also told me I was being transferred to Shands/Halifax Hospital in Daytona Beach tonight because my skin is getting worse and they cannot control it. This IVIG is more dangerous than others because it is made from human blood and has a much higher risk of complications or allergic reactions. I told him I did not want to be on this IV while in an ambulance with no doctor present in case I had a bad reaction. He finally agreed and said I will transfer tomorrow morning.

March 14, 2012

I'm still here at the same hospital in Melbourne. They say I'm being transferred every day but haven't left yet. They had me sign a transfer order yesterday but I'm still here. They say I'm going to a big hospital in Daytona Beach, Shands/Halifax 303 N. Clyde Morris Blvd. Daytona Beach, FL 32114 386.254.4000, that can handle my skin problem better.

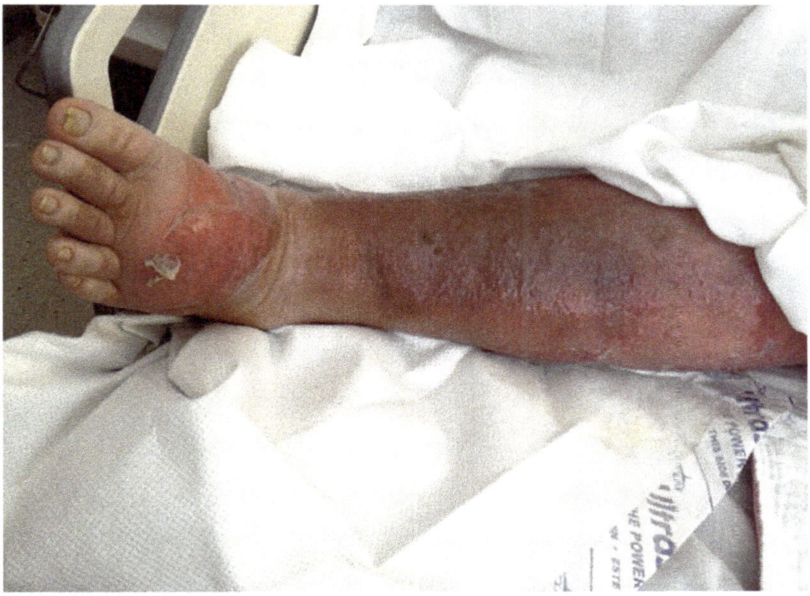

"My feet and legs feel strange today. They are getting bigger. They are swelling very much."

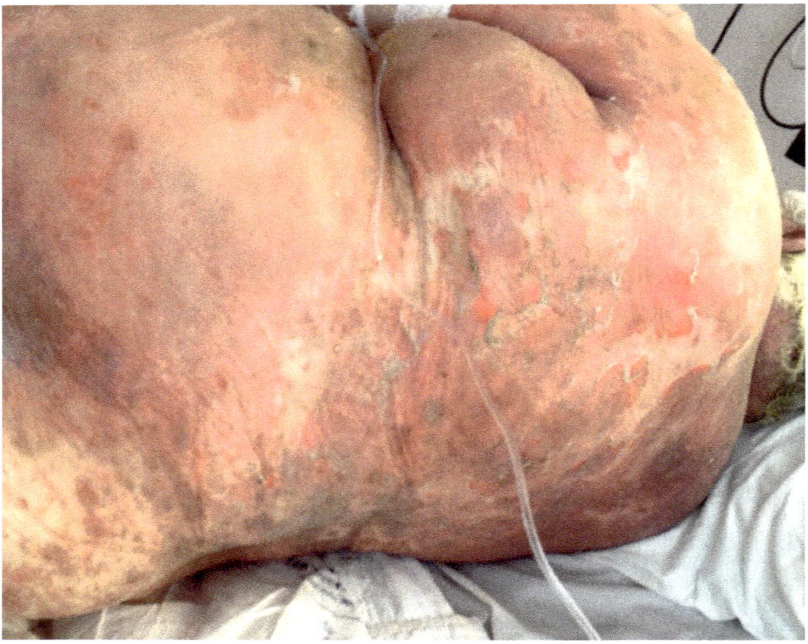

"I left a message asking for help, for prayers, for ANYTHING to stop the pain."

WAKING UP THE 'WALKING DEAD'? WHY?

Jimmie – Rant # 5

February 2020

I finally joined the Dragon Brigade in October of 2009. I was a reluctant "walking dead"! I had been in denial since January 1970. I was scared to death to have anything to do with the Veterans Administration.

In the 70's and 80's I was a professional musician living in Hollywood, CA. I spent a lot of time on Sunset and Hollywood Blvd., hanging out with a strange assortment of Vietnam Veterans.

I was around at the same time a Vietnam Veteran backed a jeep through the front door of the LA VA Hospital, in protest. Veterans existed in large numbers and made those numbers count. I took part in protests at the VA Hospital.

The few men, who understood the issues surrounding Agent Orange, were not happy with the average returning Veteran and our inability to grasp what was right in front of us. Men were already dying from Agent Orange. Spraying started on Jan 18, 1962. That is the official birthday for the Agent Orange Survivor's Club. Fifty-nine years later, no medical treatment plan whatsoever, just services on top of services, that's all you get from the Veterans Administration. And Death! The country gets two million dead Veterans. Who cares? No consideration for family health or the misery suffered all over Vietnam, and most of Southeast Asia. Google Southeast Asia, Agent Orange.

A friend who lived in Northern California at the same time told me his daughter suffered from skin rashes and the doctors could not do anything with it. That was the first time someone I served with at Phu Cat AB in 1969, expressed concern about being chemically sprayed. Still, it did not sink in.

Back in Hollywood the streets were full of homeless veterans. The VA Hospital was a huge release valve, and rallying point, from the stark poverty and stresses of daily living in the streets of Los Angeles, and when the VA turned the hospital into an armed camp, well, Veteran Nation felt betrayed. This happened in the late 1970's.

It is one thing to spit on a returning Vietnam Veteran, and call him a baby killer. But, when our government license murder against the troops, something must give. Twenty-two suicides a day or what-ever the magic number is, it's way too much giving on the part of the veteran community.

Forty years later, I could no longer deny-deny, and had to face the gauntlet of the Veterans Administration 'deny everything', do not even say the word Agent Orange. Well, Agent Orange is a fact. Two Million Vietnam Veterans are dead, and still we die. (2021).

What does it mean to be one of the 'Walking Dead'? How about rotting from the inside out.

I published my first book, "Noble Canine" on January 05, 2019, exactly fifty years since arriving at Phu Cat Air Base. I started a Blog to celebrate the 360 nights walking a Noble German Shepherd, a highly trained Sentry Dog.

At the same time, I was blogging, Medical Hemp was coming on fast and strong as dumb laws were being repealed. I challenge the VA and Governments to make Medical Hemp, Medical Marijuana and Medical Cannabis available to veterans suffering PTSD and the nerve damage done by Agent Orange. I also seek reparations for Vietnam Veterans and families. I will say it again, two million dead American Airmen, Sailors, Soldiers, Marines and Coasties. So, does this mean that the AMA/Government doctors would rather Veterans continue dying, instead of offering to the sick, pain relief from intense nerve damage caused by chemical (warfare). Instead, what we have is a safe place for better dying through fossil base chemistry, or better living through chemistry? The science and the so-called college educated professionals who created this death from the sky, are all guilty of genocide, out and out murder. You listen to me long enough you will, sooner or later, see my rage and my contempt for all USA Institutions. They all seem to end in death!

HEMP IS HEALING. The VA Pill Factories are slow death.

VA medications are oil base chemistry. This is the main reason I fear everything to do with doctors, hospitals and pharmakia, all under the auspices 'we are here to serve, and we are here to help'. What has been created by the medical cartel is the sickest country on planet earth. All the fat people of America is the first clue of just how sick a society we live in. Obesity just keeps getting younger with each generation. Surely, Reader, you have noticed fat babies.

When Agent Orange first attacked me, it went for my legs. I counted 32 falls. In the first year I went from 240 pounds, down to 165 pounds. I was dying. I got relief from nerve-pain with two medications. Pregabalin (Lyrica was its evening news name) and Tramadol (a Narcotic and a killer). When it became clear that many were dying from using Tramadol, what did my primary care doctor do? She halved my dosage. It will take longer to die. But hang in there, we will get you in the end. Isn't that special? Finally, after enough Veterans died, they changed my medication. Pharmakia is a nasty dark science.

The VA death-toll just keeps stacking up. After nine years of pills, pills, and more pills, I had no choice, I had to get away from VA oil-based chemistry, it was killing me. As far as I know, plant-based medication is not available at the VA. I needed something to replace oil-based medication which were slowly clogging the organs and keeping me tired and weak with no energy. I know this is the way it is in all of America, but it is especially true for Veterans. The medical cartel is slowly, systematically killing human beings. Wake up, this is immoral and unacceptable.

I did not know a thing about Medical Hemp. Could not understand why it was outlawed. But I made a conscience decision to find out why governments, medicine, pharmakia, corporations, and the military, the list is long, would rather watch as the citizen soldiers suffer and die and the resulting pain associated, when a simple Herb offered so much healing for a lot of problems. Two million, People! Listening? Hello!

I stopped smoking marijuana in 1986.

With the help of a Therapist/Healer, I started my search for health. Every organ in my body was chocking to death on VA oil-based medication. With herbal supplements (plant-based) and cleanses for most organs, I slowly, over an 18-month period of systematic health changes, began to feel better as the pain was under control. I started to free my body, its organs, my blood, my skin of VA toxic medication. The nerve damage done to my legs persist today. I have managed to replace VA toxic-drugs with plant-based healing. Earth plant-base healing is the only healing there is. Better living though chemistry is a lie. More 'speak-think' for a dumb-down population, by the over-educated system. There is little healing in the United States medical empire. Everything is about making money and getting patients using a long list of medication.

Hemp is the most important healing agent available on the planet. Could have saved untold amounts of pain and suffering of Vietnam Veterans, their Wives, and children.

When I confessed to my VA primary-care doctor that I was smoking marijuana again and for the first time in 33 years, her eyes smiled at me as she told me it's illegal and the Veterans Administration will never approve Hemp or Marijuana for its patients. Stupid is as stupid does. Never say never. But I wanted to be on the right side of this issue, so I signed up for the Florida State Medical Cannabis Identification Card. Get this; The state created the "Compassionate Use Registry". Isn't that a hoot? But it's a lie! There is nothing compassionate about the new state system to distribute Medical Hemp products. It's about allowing the few (mostly doctors) to get in early and, control, control baby. Boy! Do doctors and government love their two favorite words:

DENIAL and CONTROL what Monsanto (all chemical cartel(s)) and their poison products ("ROUNDUP" line) is doing to this planet is merely the tip of a big iceberg. If you think that NO SINGLE INDUSTRY CAN DESTROY THIS PLANET, THINK AGAIN. It's happening every minute of every day.

Climate change is one the symptoms and a smokescreen for a much bigger problem being covered up by media?

The 1%'s (enemies of a free-people) are so good at creating the big lie and that the big lie is that good, that adults as well as children are scared out of their minds. (Suicides, teenagers, Google). Mind control is art. Propaganda is high art. The artist who creates the will of the 1%'$ (enemies of my freedom) are master craftsmen/artist and highly sought-out and paid well to betray humankind and animalkind, while killing our home planet. Why would the too-rich (1%'$) hate humanity so much that they find it necessary to enslave the whole earth. I no longer wish to be experimented on or with. I demand all my human rights.

I demand $1,000,000/reparations for damage done during secret chemical wars of SEA/1969.

I took up smoking marijuana again in 2018.

The thirty plus years of not smoking did not prepare me for the intense highs I would experience. The pot was totally off the charts and I seldom experienced this kind of high in the past. For the first time in a long time, I experience PEACE. My pain was being controlled with Medical Hemp.

I was calmer. I could relax, now. I learned to be silent, the quiet became a sanctuary and my health thrived. To a point anyway!

I finally give my precious wife a break and needed peace, and rest from the chaos that had become our daily lives. What our women, our Veteran wives have gone through, trying to keep families together, trying to find real help for the no-name disease called Agent Orange, is an atrocity. Our care-giving wives should be compensated by the VA. Not the few hundred trickle down dollars provided by the Veterans Administration.

I demand $1,000,000/reparations for damage done during secret chemical wars of SEA/1969.

Each surviving wife and family are to share in that $1,000,000. Yes, I am calling for REPARATIONS to be paid NOW, for Vietnam Veterans and for our spouses. All 2,000,000 dead Vietnam Veterans are to be compensated, which means, that our wives and the children and the grandchildren are to be compensated. We must protect our progeny, and if not me and you, then who? Do you think for a minute that the 1%'$ controlled government and Veterans Administration gives a bloody-damn about affected generations of our children and their children as new cases of Agent Orange are now showing up, in third generation of our children?

I call on women-kind, our wives, to organize and fight for justice. Do what your able-bodied men had a chance to do but failed to do, take a stand.

Fight for full REPARATIONS OF $1,000,000 for each and every Vietnam Veteran's family. Who will stand for the children? Who will stand for the grandchildren? Most Vietnam Veterans are dying and won't be around much longer. The few surviving are sick and weary. Suicide is release from the pain of chemical warfare and the failure of VA doctors to offer any kind of treatment and healing.

My shame! While living in Hollywood, CA., I confessed to being in total denial to all things Agent Orange and its effect on the human body. I am guilty of burying my head in sand and ignoring, not facts, because government and VA never offered facts, but more and more men were dying and whole families suffering the mental anguish from chemical poisoning, was all around me. I just did not want to see it. Every Veteran from that war was intentionally kept in the dark. Lied to, cheated out of JUSTICE, cheated out of COMPENSATION.

REPARATIONS OF $1,000,000 will be paid to all surviving Vietnam Veterans and to all surviving spouses.

Either we stand together or our silence is agreement with injustice and no healing! Believe me, Vietnam Veterans are good at towing the line and shutting up. Just face the LIES! FACE all the many LIES!

When I finally entered the maze called VA services, I was excited to finally get relief from the constant pain I was in. I would meet a new face, a doctor, a nurse, technician, and I would open with 'this is caused by Agent Orange' and they, to a person, would never acknowledge my claim. (2009) It was always something else. Where is the cure? Where is the science? Why no healing in the VA system, just services to occupy our minds?

These lies, repeated over and over and over (until throw-up time) destroys the spirit to live, to struggle and fight. I observed what it did to Joseph Barbarise, my second death cause by Chemical Warfare. The first was Terry, a Marine and former Deputy. When the body rots from the inside-out, death drains via the skin, literally. The Hospice Nurses have a hard time keeping the living/dying body clean and odor free. Death has its own stench, but an Agent Orange death is the nastiest death a human can experience.

No American should ever wonder why Veterans commit suicide. Death is easier than living a lie. Betrayal by government, by AMA, and by military services, and the steady stream of lies and services coming from the Veterans Administration. But know this, all the lies are not what broke the hearts of Vietnam Veterans. Yes, the pain, the incredible pain is just too much to endure.

Too much pain watching your wife trying to deal with a husband's pain and other issues. To much pain for a man at hearing a grieving spouse crying behind closed doors. Children scared to death, watching daddy struggle and mommy falling apart. Little ones left to wonder about the future, they cry, who will take care of us?

It took the citizens who turned their backs to our problems. The pain as the American citizens turning their backs on us and abandoning a generation to our suffering and dying. As a veteran, you feel like the people would rather we just go away.

Ain't GOING TO HAPPEN!

TWO MILLION DEAD VIETNAM VETERANS, I stand for them!

GAINESVILLE, FL

Joe

March 16, 2012

They lied. They sent me to Shands Hospital in Gainesville, FL. After a week or so I was moved yet AGAIN, to Signature HealthCare Nursing Home, also in Gainesville. After about 2 weeks I told them I must have a special med called IVIG ordered by Dr. Potter from VA hospital in Tampa. I was to get this IVIG the 9th and 10th of April plus two more months. I have not gotten this med so far. Since April 11th I have been experiencing a new, big breakout of skin sores all over my arms, legs and back. I asked nurses here repeatedly to please call Dr. Potter in Tampa. I get a different answer each time. One nurse says I can't call him, then I will call, then I called but I'm waiting for his return call, then Shands hospital Dr. canceled the IVIG, then we can't do IVIG here, then we can't give IVIG on Tampa doctor's order. They keep changing their answer. Bottom line, I'm not getting the med I need that was ordered by the only doctor that seems to be able to somewhat control my problem, Dr. Potter.

April 16, 2012, the day after my birthday

I can't believe I'm 63. The doctors and nurses ordered I get a real shower every day. They've been pretty good about that, except last weekend, Saturday I believe, I had none. My skin really needs it. The next day I had a nurse I've never seen before. Very friendly, but knew nothing about me or my skin. She decided to give me a bed bath.

She found a half-used bar of soap that looked like "Irish Spring." I was the only one in the room so she assumed it was mine. She never asked she just started to use it all over me. For all other showers we used my "Head and Shoulders" for shampoo and their gold-colored liquid soap, maybe Johnson non sting soap, all over my body. At first, I hadn't felt anything, but after a minute or so it felt like my whole body was on fire. The pain was unbelievable. Not knowing what to do, I called my brother Vinny in NJ crying for help. I called the Chaplin here at this facility. He wasn't there (must have been Saturday) so I left a message asking for help, for prayers, for ANYTHING to stop the pain. The pain hadn't subsided for about 4 hours, the worst 4 hours of my life.

April 22, 2012

I'm still at Signature HealthCare in Gainesville. Last week I went to see the dermatologist and he ordered the IVIG. It's been three days and it has yet to start. I had been getting IVIG over two consecutive days in the past. This time he ordered it over three consecutive days, monthly. I pray it starts soon as the new outbreaks continue. One of my biggest fears is that one day I'll get these sores on the bottom of my feet or the palms of my hands. It's Back........ soap that looked like "Irish Spring".

May 2, 2012

I had an appointment with the Dermatologist today at the VA Hospital here in Gainesville. They are very nice there. We talked about my meds, my recovery and the IVIG meds they ordered but I have not received as yet. They said they can see improvements, but at a much slower rate than others they treated with the same disorder. They said everyone responds differently, some slower and others at a faster rate. I am the slowest so far and for unknown reasons. Instead of my main doctor being from Shands Hospital (I have no idea how that happened) they are assigning me a VA doctor as primary care so the VA will have total control of my health care. With this they feel they will be able to get the IVIG started soon. IVIG is rarely used for my condition, but they feel in my case it calls for it.

They rechecked my med list and blood test results. They said my kidney functions are a bit too high from all the meds I take. It's to be expected but needs to be watched. I asked them to be totally honest with me and my prognosis. They agreed. I am looking at a very long road ahead. I will probably never be off a long list of meds and a steady regime of skin care. My appearance will improve some, but not significantly. With the diabetes and prednisone, weight loss will be very difficult. With diabetes, my feet and legs must be watched closely to avoid amputations. That has me very worried. They are watching my lower left leg now.

Getting back to China to be with Wangli is at the top of my list of "things to do". I'm pretty sure you know that I'm about half romantic and half realist. At my age the realist part is starting to take over. I do not want to grow old alone. I also do not want Wangli to be my nurse or caregiver. I want her as a loving wife. I want to take her to dinner, buy her flowers, travel many places with her and enjoy life together as a family. I'm beginning to wonder if that will ever happen. I've had few if any fears in my life. Of those that do exist, all are related to family or lack thereof. The fear of not seeing the three most wonderful nieces in the world grow up and begin their own lives is probably a big one. Being closer to my two brothers, talking over coffee, shooting pool, playing with their dogs and especially spending Thanksgiving together. Then there is Mom. What can I say. We all love her and the fact that you never know what "mom-ism" she will utter next.

Then there are Vince, Jimmie, Willie and their wives. Unless you have spent the same moments in time with them, in the same circumstances, you just cannot know how I feel about them. We have shared experiences beyond description. We shared the happiest and the most feared, knowing we could be killed at any moment, yet we still smiled, laughed and comforted each other. When they all traveled from all over USA to come see me in Tampa hospital on the same day, I can never tell them just how much that meant to me. When Jimmie still comes to see me, when he walks in the room, I just feel energized from him being there, knowing he cares.

I've faced bad guys both while in the military and as a Deputy Sheriff. They were armed with guns, knives and assorted things they wanted to do harm to me with them. I've faced a 700 lb. tiger, a 2000 lb. rodeo bull and a few other critters that meant to do me harm, or at least lunch, but nothing as fearful, clear to the bone, as growing old alone. I'll try to keep you updated more often.

May 3, 2012

Yesterday I had an appointment to see the VA dermatologist here in Gainesville. They were not very happy at my appearance. Some skin areas improved while others declined. I told her they still have not started the IVIG that she ordered. She asked about the whirlpool bath she ordered for me. I told her there was none at Signature HealthCare, the place I was staying at. She asked if I would mind being moved to a facility or hospital wholly controlled by the VA. I readily agreed. I was moved to the Gainesville VA yesterday. Hopefully they may start the IVIG today.

The best of times, the worst of times.....!

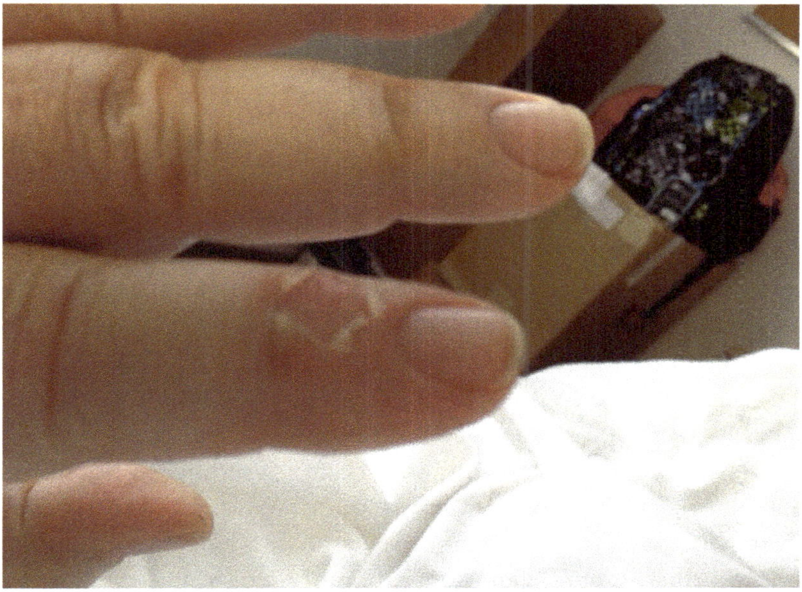

"I will probably never be off a long list of meds and a steady regime of skin care."

DOES IT MATTER WHAT WE CALL IT?
I THINK IT DOES!

Jimmie - Rant #6

1969 Phu Cat Re-Visited

I keep harping about the 2,000,000 (MILLIONs) Vietnam Veterans who have died from exposure to Agent Orange during the Vietnam War. Fifty-years later, I marvel at Veterans who seem to think attending funeral services is their calling in life. Raising money for the next memorial or honoring the Agent Orange dead and dying. When do we honor life? Death followed us home from one war, to die in a war that is even more lonely, more terrifying, so unforgiving. Wasn't enough to survive, we had to return to the world, and face man-created, body-eating death. Chemical death, a Nazi kind of death, you think. Chemical! I haven't talked about the people of Vietnam and the plague that overshadows the country. Finally, the USA is cleaning up their mess after fifty years of continued effects of chemical poisoning on the land, the animals, the people, and today, third generation new-born.

Go to Google and put in Agent Orange Vietnamese People! This is what our government is capable of. Genocide. We are governed by a sick government not of "We the People"! What has happened to the Vietnamese people and the Veterans who survived the war is not the will of an educated people. This wicked government, our government, by controlling media and education keep the citizens dumb down and ignorant. This is especially true for Veterans. I love my country, I love all the people of America, but murder by government will stop. The purpose for writing this book is to create better not change. America needs a new governmental system. The constitution died many years ago. Why? It doesn't work!

The Vietnamese people die from wounds more deadly than bullet-holes, pain just as incapacitating as any battle wound, and no one listened for fifty years. The United States is finally (?) doing the right thing with massive clean-up efforts all over Vietnam. My hope is my country does just as good a job cleaning our mess up as their professional spraying service the USAF. Vets killing vets, who would have thought, Oh! "But we didn't know!" Speed this process up, a third generation is affected and suffering. Untold numbers of Vietnamese people are dying, with many deformities. See pictures.

I did not write this book to entertain you, dear reader! All these photos are for shock-treatment only. There are thousands of pictures, all obscene, leading up to a third generation of Agent Orange victims. There are millions of real Vietnam Veterans from both sides who have simply disappeared. Died off without a word? Really! Sounds just like the 2,000,000 American Veterans of Vietnam who have died from the same chemical warfare. Most without a peep. Most not accepting GENOCIDE as their fate. Only the walking dead gets to die for the mother-lard, twice. God help my country?

Why hasn't Vietnam challenged the United States in the world Court? Does Vietnam get Justice from the United States, quietly and behind the curtain, or under the table, out of sight of accountability.

Like everything that has to do with the chemical companies (DOW, Monsanto's, DuPont and all the rest who made money off killing Americans), how do they get away with pre-meditated murder, paid for by the America people? What does the government do? Deny, deny! What does the Veterans Administration do? Deny! It's getting harder to hide 2,000,000 deaths of the home-town hero!? How many more Vietnam Veterans must die? How many of the peoples of Vietnam must suffer, die, still paying a horrible price. When does the Vietnam War end?

Dear Vietnam Veteran, here is what your government, our military and the medical cartels are doing with its cover-up of chemical warfare plague; we are being systematically destroyed, as in: suppressed, annihilated, wiped-out, wiped off the face of the earth, put a stop to, bring to an end, terminated, erased, eliminated, eradicated, obliterated, liquidated, expunged, abolished, killed, extirpated, obscured, suppressed, disrupted, rubbed-out, snuffed-out and my favorite, murdered-by-government.

Cooperate chemical producers have 'branded-together' for defense and survival of their horrid-industries products, all poisons and thrown helter-skelter to the winds on planet earth.

Our planet, our home will not survive past the two-generation warning, the allotted timeframe for repairing the earth. Sure, call me naïve, but all creatures will die out, the planet will still turn, still travel around the sun and follow the sun around the universe, but as a rock!

How can we live in a society where there is commerce without morality, or science without humanity, knowledge without character, wealth without work, pleasure without conscience, worship without sacrifice and politics without principles? It all starts with Justice. The Walking Dead demands Justice and since that is not forthcoming, this corrupt government must pay reparations.

Will somebody please tell me, how does the chemical cartel get away with their raw in your face for the world to see, murder, pray tell me? Worse yet, how do 'they' convince Vietnam Veterans to simply shut-up, lay-down and just die. It's why I am so outspoken against all Veterans groups and their refusal to confront. The only decent thing to say about Veterans Groups is the gatekeepers are dying off too, thank you Agent Orange.

I nursed two Vietnam Veterans during there long death-walk and final days in hospice. Make no bones about it, an Agent Orange death is the worst kind of atrocious death imaginable. Men's bodies so racked with pain (from the inside-out) that the Veterans Administration has special 'cocktails' to relieve pain. Those 'cocktails' are just another way to die for your country. It's necessary for this writer to be repetitive!

As Joe Barbarise lay dying in a Gainesville VA hospital/ hospice care unit, he reminded me of this fact, man, this shit (Agent Orange) was killing him, and how his life was being cut short, by 'corporate brands' and government thugs. This G.I. did not sign on for this shit! Joe did not sign on for this shit!

Joe was pissed and Joe paid a high price and Agent Orange murdered him. Another voice, silenced. The beat goes on and our numbers grow fewer each day. Just think, one of us will get the honor of being the last Vietnam Veteran to die. Who will show up at the funeral!? Who will care? Who will carry the flags!? There is always someone to blow taps!

Every day in America and from worldwide media sources, comes stories of farmers up in arms with Monsanto's and their GMO's. Chemical companies are pushing unproven technologies down the throats of a sound asleep, unsuspecting consumer. Of course, Uncle Sam is on the wrong side in this battle. A silent war to see who controls our food supply and whether the food is fit to eat. Way to go Uncle Sam!

The last ten years of my life has been about beating the Dragon to death, instead of my death. I've won, wel sort-of?! Other Veterans have battled for twenty, thirty, forty or more years. Two million have died.

So? What is wrong with this picture??

Well for one thing, that's how long we've known about the effects of the government's chemical rainbow. Agent Orange was created to destroy Vietnam the country, the Vietnamese people and the survivors who fought the war, both sides. It was a lot more than just killing vegetation. In the Court of Justice, chemical companies and the military industrial complex and government need to be adjudicated, and stopped dead in its tracks, on their planet-wide environmental destruction, OR this planet will not survive. The planet is doomed and will not survive with business as usual. The chemical cartel, the oil cartel is killing our world, our home. There is nowhere else to go.

The Veterans Administration is responsible for the biggest cover-up in all recorded history.

The whole scam, that's being played by many interested groups, be it government, media, military, or medical, is to keep Vietnam Veterans dumb down and scared. Keeps us as glorious guinea pigs with medals. It worked for fifty years. I keep returning to the central question; how many must die before a light comes on. When you suffer the pain induced by chemical warfare, the worst poison science and man can devise, and then use it as a weapon of warfare on life-itself! Agent Orange is your wake-up call. Act while you can still move!

If Vietnam Veterans had understood just how deadly the Agent Orange Plague would end up costing in lives, misery and broken families, had Vietnam Veterans stood against the chemical companies in the 1980's and stayed in the fight until victory...I am convinced, had we stopped Monsanto's, DOW, DuPont and all the rest, way back then, had we stood together, and made them pay, we could have stopped all the so-called research of GMO's at universities and corporations, stopped them cold in their tracks, and ended their reign of terror on planet earth. A lot of people are making big buck$ off our suffering and dying of Vietnam Veterans, but what chemical companies are doing with GMO's is planet-wide suicide. The end of natural farming is the end of healthy living. THEN what!?

Then, Earth will not survive 2 generations. Out-of-control oil and chemical producers will kill this planet, our home. Again folks, nowhere else to go, and Space-X will not save you.

News Flash: The Planet has warned humankind and animalkind that Earth will not support life after the next two generations. If drastic changes are not introduced worldwide, the healing of the planet will fail. The next fifty years is time enough to save our home. It won't be easy, the damage is extensive, and greed plays its game of always being in the way. In other words, the oil and chemical cartels are the problem and will not lift a hand to solve the problems they have created, unless forced to. Vietnam Veterans must be that force, even with our last breath.

Today, this May 12, 2019, the Veterans Administration is a big-time game player, playing with the lives of millions of Veterans and Vietnam Veterans. For decades, the VA has denied, denied while hundreds of thousands die. Instead of showing leadership the VA has abandoned the Vietnam Veterans and left us to die, but comfortably. Isn't that special? Sarcasm is sweet.

Agent Orange literally destroys the human body from the inside out. Seems, it goes after our legs, so most of us have difficulty standing and walking and balance is a problem. I compare Vietnam Veterans to the 'Walking Dead", as seen on TV. Hollywood has made a joke of our dilemma and made it into a drama for your viewing entertainment. They laugh all the way to the bank. The "Walking Dead" our phantoms.

Forty years ago, we were tricked by slick-as-snot lawyers who stole the needed help ($$$) that appeared to be coming forward to help Vietnam Veterans and their needy families live more comfortably. For the sick and dying Vietnam Vet, their families look on in awe and horror. These families sacrifice so much to live with one of these damaged hero's, who simply keep on dying. (TWO MILLION) I will not let you forget, dear reader.

My shame is that I allowed this holocaust of crime to happen. I never questioned my government, I just took it for granted that government was here to help me, not kill me. Big mistake! I trusted Doctors and I was thankful for the VA. Never again.

VA HOSPITAL, GAINESVILLE, FL

Joe

May 8, 2012

I have been feeling pretty bad for some time. The pain has been pretty bad. I've been getting sad all the time, having serious doubts about ever getting back to China to marry Wangli. I keep reading all I can find about my illness and the meds involved. Three days ago, they restarted me taking that IVIG special med for my skin condition. All medical web sites state that skin improvements, though it doesn't always help, may begin in 1-2 days or as long as 3-4 weeks. The hospital arranged for me to get 5 days in a row of this med (at $10,000 per day) taking 6-10 hours each day. After the first day several people stated I looked better. I considered they say that to make me feel better mentally. I had no new sores that day, but occasionally I would have a day sore free.

The second IVIG day I was again new sore free and I thought I felt slightly better. More nurses commented about me looking better. I actually felt a little better for sure. The third IVIG day came and I knew for sure I was feeling a lot better. No new sores for three days and the old ones drying and clearing. My mental attitude much improved. Now I can see the light at the end of the tunnel. I can see my goals. They are possible.

That same morning my friend Jimmie arrived to see me. He was shocked how well I looked and sounded. We were laughing and joking. I had not laughed in so long a time. It felt great. Vince called at the same time and we were all feeling great. Vince, Jimmie and I got along great. I draw a lot of energy from Jimmie and Vince. It almost feels like drugs I feel so good.

That lasted a couple of hours until......

All of a sudden, I was feeling bad. It was hard to breathe. When you can't get your breath, that's panic time. Jimmie got the nurse. One look at me and she grabbed the oxygen for me then called the doctor. The IVIG puts massive amounts of fluid into my body. One side effect could be pneumonia, fluid build-up in my lungs. Another possible side effect is blood clots in legs, lungs or elsewhere.

After about an hour they took me off the Oxygen and I felt better. The doctor sent me to get a CT scan of my chest to check for pneumonia. If I lay flat on my back, my obese stomach pushes up against my diaphragm causing breathing difficulties. The opening of the CT scan device is also quite small and causes claustrophobic feelings in many people. The techs made me lay back almost flat, raised my arms over my head and tried to cram me into a clearly too small opening. The breathing became difficult again. I felt like sardine number 15 trying to be crammed into a can for 12. A little yelling later and I was removed from the CT scan and placed on O2 again. My best day became my worst, BUT, I can now still see the light at the end of the tunnel. I now believe again that my dreams of China, Wangli and marriage are a real possibility and I will keep working for those goals.

Today and tomorrow are my last two IVIG days for another month. The doctors said they will start looking for another nursing home/rehab facility to send me at that time. I'm not sure exactly where or when.

It's 11AM and the doctor just left. He told me I had a staph infection in my blood and he has me on IV antibiotics for that. He thinks it's from when my Pemphigus went septic (severe blood poison) twice in China.

SURVIVAL

Jimmie - Rant #7

Surely, dear reader, you can feel or sense Joe's will to live. The pull of China, Nurse Wangli and the English students at university, the orphans, all pulled at his heart and it gave him hope. Hope that the VA was on the right track, and at the end of the tunnel was a lighthouse, pointing westward.

This nonsense about moving Joe to a rehab nursing center is insanity. As soon as Joe shows any sign, whatsoever of doing better, improving, if it looks like Joe is going to 'make-it', the VA and its excuse for doctors are again ready to ship him to somewhere, as soon as they find a medical facility willing to enter the twilight zone of unanswerable questions, main one being; 'Why is the Veterans Administration pushing responsibility for Joe's medical care out to lesser hospitals who are nowhere ready to deal with the number of issues in Joe's portfolio.' The medical establishment was not prepared to offer any kind of treatment. No hospital in North America has any experience dealing with the effects of chemical warfare.

While VA doctors denied the reality of Agent Orange, the American medical cartel has protected the oil and chemical cartels for the past hundred plus years. At the same time, two million Veterans died, much like Joe suffered and died. For fifty years Vietnam Veterans were dying like flies, while responsible adults denied, denied that Agent Orange was responsible for any deaths. While VA doctors denied the ravages, VA office slugs were hard at work denying benefits.

Not only did veterans suffer, but whole nations were affected by the chemical warfare raged on Vietnam and most of southeast Asia. The veteran, his wife and his children were left to their own devices which means they suffered alone, most in poverty. Two million dead G.I.'s, just a bunch of nobodies, who suffered just like Joe did.

'Fuck it, don't mean a thing, move on!' Is a damn lie!

Why do most Veterans not join veteran's organizations. Those that do join are soon disappointed by the non-direction all the Veterans groups seem to wander around in. I was. We stay home! Sorry to say it, but the VVA's slogan of no future generation of Veterans will be left behind, is pathetic. But it's quite OK sweeping Agent Orange under the rug. It's the main reason I don't attend any meetings of an organized veteran group. Half the men who join sit at home on meeting night, wondering where the voice for Veterans is hidden.

We can't receive Hemp oil products for medication purposes via VA, because of ignorant laws, and ignorant doctors. We pay with our lives! Bad law that has cost two million Vietnam Veterans their lives. If it were anybody else, you'd hear words like holocaust or genocide. Two million airmen, sailors, soldiers, marines and coasties, plus family members of the infected. New and the latest survey from the VA is, 'how many of your children's children are affected by Agent Orange poisoning.' And dare we discuss the effect suffered upon the people and animals and land of Vietnam the country.

My own story: I was forced by Agent Orange to apply for Veterans benefits, and at the same time, Social Security Disability.

The Disabled American Veterans (DAV) became my champion and advocate with all things VA and getting access to what's due to me and all veterans of the Vietnam War.

"Noble Canine Search for the Edge" took me ten years, from starter outline to finished product to write and publish.

During the ten years it took to write Noble Canine my body was being decimated and beaten to death by chemical poisoning and the painful acknowledgement realizing and accepting a cruel betrayal of this country. This has never happened before. Google the 'bonus Army' of World War One. They too were betrayed and lied to.

During the first three years battling this disease, nerves were attacked, muscles attacked, skin attacked. Loss of appetite. Loss of 60+ pounds in three months. I felt the cold breath of death. Finally found some pills that relieved the pain, but I continued to fall a lot. Most were embarrassing falls in embarrassing places.

It took several years for the affected nerve and muscle damage to spread from my lower left leg, all the way up to the hip, then cross-over or through the hips to the right leg and travel all the way down to the toes. My nerves endings in my legs were so damaged, I started wishing for a wheelchair.

If I didn't start eating again, and lots of protein, I may never want to eat again. So, I forced myself to eat a big breakfast and added beans and rice from my favorite chicken house, and it stopped the weight loss. That was a huge victory for me. Of course, I gained weight. I also recovered all my lost weight and then some. I was so weakened by nerve damage that I was unable to regain any muscle strength or to bulk up. I went from overweight, to skinny as a rail to fat again. All the while just under my skin a raging fire burned, like thousands of fire ants, feasting on my nerves and muscles and skin. Relentless pain!

I thanked the VA gods for the pain-free hours of relief the pills palace was providing.

Over the 10 years of writing, I went from intense pains to mild pains, and finally completed my book, 'Noble Canine, Search for the Edge'. For three years I didn't lift a pen, or turn on a computer. I just set still, and gave my body the desire to live. I want to be a part of the book's success. Lovely stories are already coming out of the woodwork. During the ten years it took to write the book, I watched two Noble Warriors succumb to the ravages of Agent Orange and die in Hospice Care. Horrible deaths. Nobody should have to live a life of the walking dead!? Vietnam Veterans are the 'Walking Dead'! Not the TV crap.

Worse, I use to go to veterans' meetings and it is always the same. Someone just died from Agent Orange, or is so sick, and is in a hospital and will soon die. Every meeting hall in America will tell the same story of cold death, lonely death, wasn't supposed to happen like this. I survived the Vietnam War, I made it home in one piece. But now, after ten years of being in the fight to live, I have seen our demons, and I fight to control my hate. The 'Walking Dead' will not go silently into the dark. Not this one anyway!

Hemp Oil is a healing gift from the Creator. Still the VA turns a blind eye to pain and suffering and the healing power that is Hemp. It makes no sense to me. The medical establishment is dead to healing. The smile of death is their calling card. I am fixated of death and dying and the horrors of chemical warfare, but what else is there?

Why are Hemp products denied to Veterans? Why is that, President Trump? Why is that, President Biden? Why, as commander in chief of our military, do you reject the healing power of Hemp Oil. Pill Palace Pharmakia is based on old world oil. Hemp Oil is New Earth and healing! Let's hear it for plant-base healing. I am a believer.

Mr. President, with all due respect for the office, stop the 22 suicides daily. Two Million Vietnam Veterans have suffered enough and paid with their lives, all the while being told no problem, GI? Lies kill. VA kills, governments kill and I struggle to be composed.

Law Enforcement needs to get out of the hemp business. Law enforcement, along with politicians, and governments have done much damage to the veteran community, our citizens and the America psyche. President Biden, your continued non-support of the military is cheapened and hypocritical to the office. Veterans are tired of the machine of government. Maybe it is time to make a big change in representative government. Most Veterans will not play the games. Stop denying this miracle-wonder-working-powerful plant from our Creator. Supply free Hemp products to aid the veteran. The VA should just pretend hemp is just another pill to be served up in massive dosage. The best medical experience is a healing experience. Heal our people? The government must stop killing its own people. Make medical hemp oil available to a sick society. The Planet is sick and dying. We either heal the planet and heal our bodies, or we all become memories. Just another rock flying through space. Save the planet?

VA HOSPITAL, GAINESVILLE, FL

Joe

May 8, 2012 (continued)

It's now 2 PM same day. Busy day today. Two doctors were here and just left. They were very concerned. It seems my staph blood infection is rather serious. One of the doctors was from dermatology and the other from infectious disease. Both my problems, the staf and the Pemphigus, are very serious. Both require a different approach for containment. Fighting one, increases the other one. If they treat the staph, it makes the Pemphigus come back again much worse. If they continue to fight the Pemphigus, it strengthens the staph blood infection. They went to consult with other doctors and will come back soon today to let me know their plan. Last time this happened in China I was in a coma three days. While we talked, I got the strong impression how concerned they were about the seriousness of all this. I could feel how serious it is to choose between which illness do they attack and which do they let run wild, as the treatments are totally opposite. I'm worried. I'll let you know more a little later.

It's now 4pm and three more doctors just left after a long conversation with me. I'll try to shorten it. FACT: A staph infection did for sure show up in the both vacuum blood bottles they used on me yesterday and day before, one on each arm. It is very serious and can be fatal.

FACT: everyone has many bacteria all over their body on the outside. It's normal and usually not a problem.

FACT: Many people, myself and most health care workers, have a form of antibiotic resistant, or super-staph, in their nose called MRSA.

FACT: those vacuum blood drawing tubes are filled with exactly their name....vacuum. Upon insertion into the skin, they immediately suck in, not expel outward. The phlebotomy is what draws the blood is supposed to rigorously clean the skin surface where they will draw the blood using a special cleaning tool. They must rub very hard and for at least 30 seconds. On normal skin it may hurt a little. On me it feels like you are holding a fire to my skin causing extreme pain.

FACT: There are two ways that the staph infection got into that vacuum tube. #1-it was in my blood and drawn into the tube (very bad). #2-the skin was possibly not pre cleaned good enough, due to the extreme pain and me yelling loudly, and the bacteria was sucked into the vacuum tube "off" my skin and not from in my blood and into the vacuum tube (much better).

How to choose between two equally horrific options?

What else? We called Las Vegas and asked for Jimmy The Greek, world famous odds maker, and asked him to give us the odds on either pick. He thought a few moments then said, "Sorry Joe but this one is even too close for me to call. Your only option is my time honored SDF." So, his right hand slid deep into his pocket and pulled out a well-worn, 1923 silver dollar. With a flick of his wrist, that coin soared into the air flipping end over end as it's done on many occasions for him. I heard him clearly say, "Heads we fight the pemphigus or tails we fight that staph blood infection." I had Jimmy The Greek on speaker phone so the doctors and I could clearly hear. The coin fell to a carpeted floor, bounced one time before landing. Jimmy The Greek softly said, "It's heads facing up Joe. Are you ready for your fight?" I told him I was ready for the fight for my life. I was armed well. I prayed every day. My family prayed for me and had their extended family, friends and church/ecclesia members pray for me too. He softly said, "I wish you well" as he hung up the phone.

That's how we chose to bring the fight to Pemphigus, let the staph infection slide, and see in a few days if we chose well. Stay tuned right here for the continuing drama "Choices", starring Joseph Barbarise and Jimmy the Greek. Co-starring the entire staff of Gainesville Florida V.A. Hospital. Brought to you from Florida.

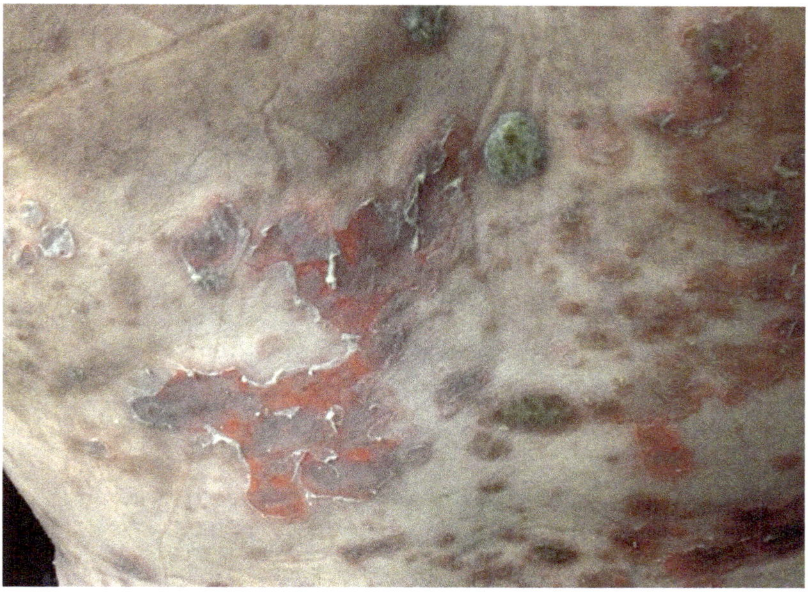

"I never thought I would deteriorate so quickly. I'd swear I had many more years left in good health."

FRIEND TO CELEBRITIES

Jimmie - Rant #8

Joe was an A#1 photographer. Joseph Barbarise was well known around the rich and famous, a small circle of friends which included Jimmy the Greek of Las Vegas fame. Shaquille O'Neal was a friend of Joe's. Joe took much joy telling of their meetup in China and being invited to lunch with the great basketball player. They both lived in Orlando, Florida for a while.

Joe had an exceptional good eye for AnimalKind. He took daring photographs. Several times he danced with death trying to get the perfect photo. His favorite stories involving a tiger and a big ass bull.

I will share a story from our nights together in Vietnam. Nights were mostly the same, night after night, it got dark and our enemies were happy. Most nights you worked alone, with your dog. Vietnam was a lonely and deadly place and dark time was the VC and NVA's playground. So, the work of clearing a post the size of a football field was dangerous. Some nights you got a break and spent the long night in the company of the dog team on the next post to you. Someone to talk to, and it was a big deal. Joe and I were on the short side of our 365-night tour. We often met on each other's post and spent a few hours bullshittin'. This night Joe will be coming my way, and I was interested in all things having to do with his girlfriend in Qui Nhon. Joe was sneaking off base to go see her, putting his life in danger, a big-time no-no, as in a LBJ moment. Never slowed him down. But tonight, it was different. Well before midnight Joe and Prince showed up and Joe is dragging his bucket along. After settling in he opens his bucket and pulls out a tiny portable TV. Next, he set up a little cook stove, started a fire and began to heat up and pop popcorn. The smell was intoxicating, and the popping was incredibly loud, and we wondered what the VC were thinking, and the Cobra Flight guards were thinking in their bunkers. The last two items Joe pulled from his bucket were two warm beers. With VC listening and wild animals listening and the bunker and tower guards listening, Joe and I enjoyed our little party in war-torn Vietnam.

Joe had a playful sense of humor.

Oh! One other thing, Joseph's contact via phone with Jimmy the Greek, well, let me put it this way, I ain't going to tell! Did it happen or not?

VA HOSPITAL, GAINESVILLE, FL

Joe

May 9, 2012

At 5:30 this morning, for no apparent reason I just woke up. It was still dark outside. I just lay there in the quiet darkness. About 6:00 AM someone opened the door a little and asked if she could come in. I agreed. It was a nurse named Claudette, someone I never met before. I asked her what she wanted and she said God told her to meet and talk with me.

It seems her husband has a disease a little similar to mine with the sores and extreme pain. She felt I needed someone to talk with, someone to pray with. I was completely shocked. We talked and prayed about a half hour. I felt a little better. Before leaving, she took my vital signs. My temperature was normal. No sign of infection. BP and sugar levels a bit high but it's caused by all the meds I take. No nausea, vomiting, dizziness or any other sign of infection.

May 9. 2012

Well, another day is coming to an end. Sunny and almost 90 degrees.

It was beautiful here, or so I'm told. I was busy waiting for my vital signs to change, to say whether I had that staph blood infection they told me about yesterday or not. So far, no signs. Temperature normal and no other signs showing. Maybe that coin flip yesterday was right. It looks like I'll probably be here until Monday while they look for the next place to send me and keep looking for those signs of infection. Wish me luck.

May 11, 2012

It's 3 PM and my nurse just walked in, the phlebotomist that will draw blood cultures to retest for staph blood infection. It takes three days to complete the test so,I guess no real results until at least Monday.

My case worker was just here. She is the one looking for another facility to take,me. She said she applied to several that turned me down. She will start to call all of them in Orange, Seminole and Brevard counties to look for somewhere for me.

Have you ever wondered..........?

Still May 11, 2012

Good news, good news and a little bit of bad news.

It seems that after the blood culture test, they can get a prelim result in one day and that result is almost always correct. My prelim just came back positive for the blood born staph infection. The nurse didn't want to tell me but when I saw her try to start a new antibiotic on me, I made her.

I swear I was going crazy. I just couldn't catch a break. I told her I wanted to talk with the Chaplin tomorrow and the doctor now. I then called my brother Anthony and had him put Vinny on conference call so we all could hear the same thing at the same time in case I really was going crazy.

The doctor could tell I was distraught. I told him about the blood cultures and he, Dr. Du, said he knew and already ordered yet another blood culture and could not get it until Monday. He said the first three being positive it's highly likely number four will be positive too. He did not know why the other doctors told me they could not treat both staph and Pemphigus at the same time but it was not true. They can do both. They will do both.

About half hour ago the nurse started an antibiotic to start fighting the staph. Dr. Du stated they already rescheduled another round of IVIG in 2-3 weeks to continue fighting Pemphigus. The bad news is that I probably do have the staph infection and it takes

4-6 weeks to overcome. The good news is it is curable. In 4-6 weeks, the staph will be gone and my skin should be the best it's been in 2 years.

It's about 5 AM and as usual I just can't sleep well. I keep waking up every 20-30 minutes sometimes with a crazy dream and other times for unknown reasons. I have to say that after talking to Dr. Du yesterday with my brothers on conference listening, I do feel better, less stressful. It's not all gone mind you, but much better. Yesterday I asked for a consult (meeting) with the Chaplin today. Even after talking with Dr. Du I still just "feel" like I must. I talked via email earlier with my friend Jean Whitt. She prayed for me and I'm not sure but I'm starting to think she has a "red phone" or hotline to the "big guy" upstairs. The good news started coming soon after that. My skin continues to visibly improve daily.

May 12, 2012

Saturday. Have you ever wondered what you would do if you came face to face with your own mortality? Imagine if you had three whole days and nights with nothing to do at all but think....... think about finding out in the next three days if you would literally live or die. You could watch TV, but didn't want to. You could surf the Internet for anything known to mankind, but couldn't concentrate more than a few moments. You could call any friend or family member but were afraid of having mood swings making simple conversation all but impossible.

This is what I'm facing right now. I had the newest blood cultures drawn yesterday. Now they must sit for three days until sometime Monday to give us the answers. There are two different types of answers. The doctors will look for simple answers, either negative or positive. That is the scientific approach. The other, more human approach is what either scientific answer really means. If the culture comes back positive it means I have a staph blood infection which could probably kill me in the not-so-distant future. If it comes back negative it means there is no staph infection. It means the other test was a double false positive and I will probably not die so soon, in fact it means I will probably be well enough to return to China later this year, marry Wangli and live a pretty happy life.

Waiting, waiting, waiting. So hard to concentrate. So hard to think of anything else.

May 16, 2012

Here it is........2 AM and I just woke up. I'm still in Gainesville V.A. Hospital but just can't sleep. I keep waiting for any day now that Social Services from this hospital will walk in here telling me I'm moving right now to some other facility in unknown location.

I keep thinking about returning to China. The big problem is the IVIG med I take for the Pemphigus and its cost. In order for me to have this med in China, I need approval from the Chinese Central Government and about $6,000 a day. It could be from 2-5 days in a row, so add hospital costs too. Here in USA, I get the IVIG like last month, 5 days in a row. It costs $10,000 per day here. That's $50,000 for only one month treatment. I cannot afford that.

We are looking for some Chinese meds that do the job of IVIG. I wrote to Dr. Dong asking her to try to visit a Korean hospital in Kaifeng that specialize in skin disorders. I want her to try to find Chinese meds that will take the place of IVIG so I can return to China.

One of the nurses just walked in carrying hot water so I can make instant coffee. She is very nice. Nurse shift changed here at 2 AM.

May 16, 2012, 2:30 PM

Social services were just here. She told me she is still looking, but so far has found no facility willing to take me in. Nursing homes and rehabs are not in business to make money.

May 16, 2012, 3:30 PM

The Ultrasound techs just left. They did a DVT test on my left leg looking for blood clots. Maybe I'll get the results later today. My legs are swollen the last few days, most especially the lower left one. I couldn't see it but the tech said its so big that it's seeping fluid all over. It's very painful to the touch.

May 17, 2012

Doctors, nurses and CNA's have been in and out of here. Results of DVT test are in. No blood clots in my legs. That's both good as well as a little bad news.

No clots as good news: There are no clots to suddenly break loose, travel to my heart or lungs, and, well, you can guess. They DO know how to treat blood clots.

No blood clots as bad news: They have no idea what's wrong with my legs, why they are so VERY swollen and painful to the touch, why they are oozing lots of fluid through the skin, or what to do about it. My left leg has gotten so big the last two days that I can't even lift it. Some of my friends and family cannot understand how the doctors can be puzzled. What I have is so rare, no one has ever seen this before. They don't know what to do.

Sunday May 20, 2012

It's about 11 PM and I don't know what to do. The pain in my left calf is really bad. More by the hour. I called the nurse and told him. He is very kind and tries his best. He gave me whatever pain meds I had available and tried to position my left leg so the calf is almost not touching the bed. I can't imagine how it will feel in a few weeks or even a few more days. My movements are getting less and less. The pain is getting more again. I keep sliding down in the bed. Yesterday they got four nurses to grab a pad under me on each corner and drag me higher up towards the headboard as I had no strength to do that myself. They did not have enough people here to try that again tonight. They have to put me on oxygen more and more to get my breathing under control. I'm on it now for at least the third time today.

11:45 PM Would you want to know???

If you had the chance to be told which day, which hour would be your last opportunity to do something, be it dancing with your wife, eating regular food, using the toilet alone or simply not in great pain......you want to know? I mean really?? I never thought I would deteriorate so quickly. I'd swear I had many more years left in good health to be with Wangli in China. We would do all those things I wanted to do with her, including traveling around China together.

Now, day by day I can feel my body slipping away, getting weaker. My friends and family tell me as I would tell them to stay strong, don't give up, you will get better again, believe in God. He can do anything. I try, I really do, but I'm not sure how much I really do believe. I pray I'm wrong and I have a long time left, but I'm not sure, not sure I even want to.

I can't imagine being stranded in bed, unable to get up, more pain every day.

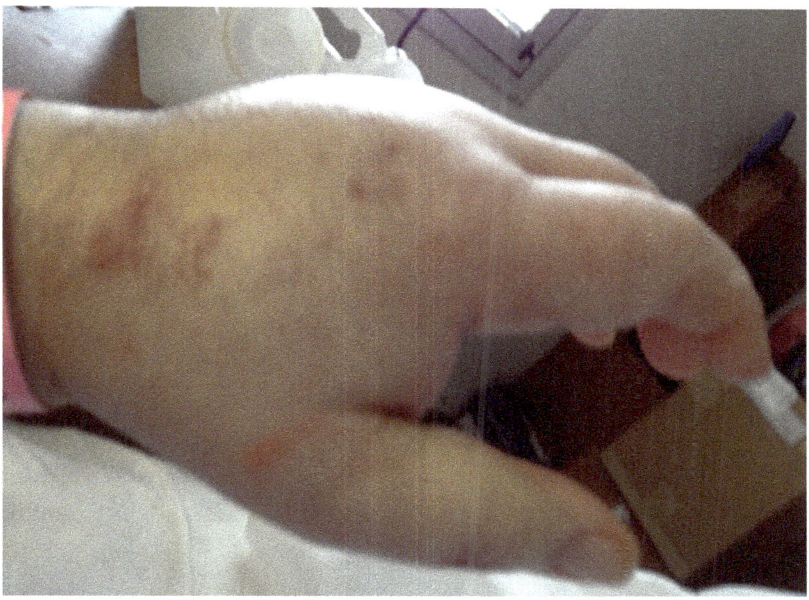

"... very swollen and painful to the touch."

THE GOOD, THE BAD, AND THE UGLY

Jimmie - Rant #9

1969 Phu Cat Re-Visited

December in Vietnam is all about going home. Ten days till Christmas, and all I know is in 20 days and a wake-up I'll be back in the world. A place with fewer eyes with hate in them is all I hoped for. I have 19 more working nights with my Noble Canine, Junior, a mighty dog if there ever was. In fact, a MWD Hero. I got Junior after his handler was severely wounded being ambushed taking that first step into the twilight zone. See "Noble Canine, Search for the Edge", pet lovers for the rest of the story.

One thing I've noticed about Christmas 2019, fifty years later, 'they're' not beating up on the meaning behind Christmas since Mr. Trump took over governing the American Swamp. Is President Trump a good President or a bad President? 'Frankly my dear, I don't give a damn'.

The Presidency: Obama or Trump or Clinton, the Bushes, even, god forbid it, even Ronald, ALL CREATED AND OWNED BY 1%'s. In the end, President Trump does as he is told, same-same for all past presidents. As far as the future is concerned, it will be business as usual unless we stand against the injustice and hate of the 1%'s.

Life on Planet EARTH is ending, not earth!

The Earth does not need to be a barren rock just because some questionable human-types hate earthlings. The 1%'$ greed is the root of this evil. In fact, the only evil caused anywhere in this world is created by 1%'$ to keep us all in line, enslaved, all of humanity in chains.

The 1%'$ created 'The Matrix' the movie, to boast of the con-job done on the world.

So, us simpletons, we the people, wanting only to be entertained, we go to the theater, upgrade to a tub of (GMO) popcorn with lots of grease and a super-size coke and give alms of pleasure and praise to Hollywood for producing such a creative story of our own slavery. The story of our slavery is creative propaganda, and this comes from the art community. Lies on top of lies and so much misinformation, that no wonder stress is a killer. The artist/creators who serve the 1%'$ make Hitler's artist/creators look like schoolgirls. The 1%'$ love to boast, so 'see you at the movies' should have special meaning. Don't be afraid to look. It's part of our destiny to be overcomers.

All this verbiage just to point out and let you in on a secret, that you, we, me, do not decide who will be the next President of the USA. You get to vote and play 'drain the swamp' using computers to count our votes. We the people, lose! Every Presidential election is creative bait and switch and fraud. 1%'$ choose the candidates of both parties and we get to choose the lesser of two evils. Some choice? The biggest mistake and coup de grace in voting is using computers to count the vote. The big lie shoved down our throats that paper ballots are slow and cumbersome and take too much time to count. Lies.

Paper ballots vs computers. Well, most Americans own at least one computer, and how has that worked out for you. Computers are trouble and intrusive. As long as they work, we ignore their controlling of our lives. As long as your computer is up and running, we look the other way. Computers must be continually updated. They have a short life span. Tech companies keep the consumer in a void of ignorance. It makes no difference if you're young and computer smart you still are a subject to the computer. The computer age is fresh and new and aids slavery. Consider this: every click you make eventually leads to creating income streams. Ten dollars here, thirty dollars there and the cost just keeps going up and the apps (toys) become burdens.

Nothing about computers justifies removal of our rights as free citizens.

THE GOOD THE BAD AND THE UGLY

Of course, I'm talking about the Veterans Administration.

The Good:

Finally, after 10 years of being locked-in with the VA, they did something, that had the hint of healing in it. The VA awarded Brooks Adaptive Sports a grant to provide for Veterans, opportunities to be involved in sports. Brooks provides for special needs which is something nobody does better. Some of the activities for Veterans are cycling, yoga, rowing, skeet shooting, fishing, and basketball.

I've been trying to get the VA to provide access to swimming that would strengthen my weakening body, especially my legs and this has gone on for years. I was hoping to use the pool at the Brooks/YMCA and have the VA pick up the expense. Instead, the VA wanted me to travel to Lake City VA or the Gainesville VA. I even found a church with an indoor-heated pool. On the day I visited, there were 3 or 4 veterans in the pool, all were doing therapy. The people in charge told me just what I needed to do, a no brainer, right? Wrong! My primary doctor refused, again.

Why is swimming so important?

After Agent Orange decimated my legs, making walking and balance issues, requiring a four-wheeled walker, I was scared I was going to lose the use of my legs. I didn't want to end up in a wheelchair. I realized that if I didn't find some way to exercise my legs, rebuild strength which would improve my balance, I might be wheelchair bound.

But in 2019 something happened that offered real hope and the VA was not the originator, as their usual, but Brooks Rehabilitation came to my rescue.

I walk and exercise at a softball park in the neighborhood with a half mile walking track/parking lot. I'm walking to save my legs. I fear if I don't use them, I will lose them. If I could make one trip around the half-mile circle, I was doing good. Sometimes I could make it around twice, that was an exceptionally good day for me.

But one morning while walking, I encountered cyclists, lots of odd-looking cycles. People were almost lying on their backs and flying around the park. This is the first time I understood the term recumbent. Bikes or Trikes are three-wheeled and recumbent. If you couldn't use your legs, Brooks had hands-only peddles and recumbent. If unable to use hands, pedals for the feet, sticking out in front of the Trikes. I was in shock; I had never seen so many Trikes.

I can do this. I can do this! Yes, do you sense my excitement? The riders were having fun. I'm sure I can do this. I talked to the Brooks rep and found out I could be out riding, as part of a new VA effort to reach out to the Veteran community. I got myself signed up and enjoyed my first Saturday morning ride at the large Blue Cross & Blue Shield campus.

I was hooked and I knew I could do this and that these trikes are the answer to rebuilding muscle and strength and saving the use of my legs.

Was I happy? Oh yeah! Big time. The Brooks people had a contact at the VA whose sole job was helping Veterans acquire the three-wheeled-recumbent cycles. It took three months, recording my activities, keeping track of the exercises I was doing. Where it stands now, today…I'm waiting for the VA/ Prosthesis Department to evaluate and approve the diagnosis which, if okayed, will free the monies for purchasing a brand-new trike, built especially for Jimmie Moore. I am so excited. Come on VA, please get it right this time.

Beside cycling, I'm rowing and trying to do yoga.

The rowing is another exercise that really builds strength and goes hand-in-hand with cycling. I've accomplished my first 15-mile ride on a recumbent bike. I feel there is no limit to how far cycling can take me. I've become the poster child for Brooks Adaptive Sports and Recreation. Thanks Brooks People! Soon I will do a blog about Brooks Rehabilitation. They are the most caring people on the planet. The ten years I've battled Agent Orange, Brooks Rehab is a big reason I'm doing as well as I am.

For years I was helped and healed by Brooks. I did both Physical and Occupational Therapies at Brooks, for years. Brooks is about healing.

The Bad:

Until I got so sick, really sick, I didn't want anything to do with the Veterans Administration.

I had no choice. Outside the VA, Doctors don't know what Agent Orange is or how to come up with a treatment plan. Guess what? Neither does the VA. Fifty years of denials, no real health care, just the facade of doing. Do you need an ear-piece? Or glasses? Or surgery on your eyes? The VA is there for you? Medication? Oh my god, medication out the ass. Feet a problem? No problem, the VA got you covered.

Once you get in the systems and you're issued your beanies, the facade comes tumbling down and the Veterans, sooner or later, understands there is no healing to be found in the crowded halls of the VA infrastructure.

Here's the thing that make me angry, I keep seeing Veterans with legitimate claims not able to get a penny. If the system doesn't provide healing, then what is the real purpose of VA Health Care. Veterans cannot purchase the medical help they need, and they suffer. Mainly they just die.

VA protocols are rigged in favor of providing nothing.

Most Veterans will not play this game. I went to the VA because I had no alternative. But when I talk to warriors from the Vietnam War and hear their tales of woe, I can see their suffering. It's real. It's a narrow path for the walking dead. We have no friends.

I'll say this for Vietnam Veterans, we know how to suffer.

Our spouses are our care givers, and they suffer and fight to give a normal life to their husbands and family. The government murdered us, after betraying us. The VA has lied for 50 years. The family and friends that surround a veteran are all they have, and most of the time the families do not understand what's going on. People just don't get it when it comes to what the real pain is all about.

The Ugly:

Not allowing access to medical Hemp, medical Cannabis, medical Marijuana. Planned Genocide! Murder by government. Thank you, Mr. President and Commander in Chief.

I STAND, EVEN IF ITS ALONE...

VA HOSPITAL, GAINESVILLE, FL

Joe

Monday May 21, 2012

It's about 5:00 AM. I just had a bowel movement. Such an embarrassing event. With my left leg feeling numb, it's time for bed pans. I hate them. Nurses do too as big as I am, I do too. Most nurses and assistants here are very understanding. A few are not. Al argues and seems to think I'm faking. My left leg just won't move. I tell him to please pull the sheets slowly and it hurts much slower and it hurts much less. Pull faster and it hurts MUCH more. He always pulls faster. I asked him to please check my catheter. He doesn't even look, just says over and over, it's ok, it's ok. If it falls off, I will urinate all over the bed.

It's been two days now and no cream meds or Vaseline applied to my back or skin. My hands are shaking more. When I woke up the oxygen was on my face. I'm really worried. I'm getting the feeling I'll never leave here.

The nurse just came in to check my cath. Said there is sediment in it showing my kidneys are working too hard. It's a sign of septic (not good).

About 8 AM (it's 9:45 now) a special nurse came in named Mae. She is so kind. A Filipino-American nurse in charge of PICC lines as special IV points. She puts them in and maintains them. It's a specialty. Wangli called at same time. What this nurse does causes me extreme pain. I tried to hide from Wangli but could not, especially after I made a Chinese exclamation "teng teng" which means pain, pain. She knew I was hurting.

After that I received a call from unexpected person. My Aunt Mae called. She is the best one in Barbarise family. My mom even likes her. Her and Uncle Dominick are the greatest people.

A new nurse (to me) was here this morning named Freddie. Nice guy. He gave me more info. I had an external cath for a few days. Yesterday when I passed out, they installed an internal-cath. They also tried sternum rub to wake me. No good.

It takes very little to really make me happy. Different things from different people. Jeff is the busiest person I know. From him, it's just the time to call me.

Vinny and Anthony: both, just a call or visit. Both very busy. I love them both.

Mom: wellllllllll..... I can say a phone call or I can say with a smile, one less call:-)) She is great but cannot understand time differences or rest.

George: he never calls but never misses a chance to talk to me. It's the sound of his voice. I know we met only once but I can tell he cares. It's that sound from him.

Wangli: a slight hint of a tear OR a smile from her. Either will do. I can hear both.

Jimmie and Virginia: the sound of true caring. It's always there.

Vince: the sound of "it's a minor thing, don't worry, you'll be well soon.". I know it's bull**** but he almost makes me believe it too.

Will: (my best male friend in China) the sincere sound of miss you, wish you were here again, wish you never left, love you.

Candy: (my best female friend in China) the sincere sound of miss you, wish you were here again, wish you never left, love you.

Willie: just him in general. His friendliness. It's in his voice but indescribable. His wife very similar. I guess he found someone as nice as he is. I'm very happy he did.

FACTS ARE STARING US DOWN

Jimmie - Rant #10

April 29, 2020

Facts are Staring Us Down!

The obvious solution to keeping Vietnam Veterans Organizations up and running is in the hands of our Agent Orange Surviving Wives. In five years, most VFW's and VVA's (all Vet orgs.) will be headed by and ran by the brides of Vietnam Veterans. I can see it now, VVA becomes VVAW, and that is how our voice and our spirit will continue into the near future. Much thanks to our Women, our Brides.

I must have been exposed while hanging out with hundreds of Vietnam Agent Orange victims along with their wives at the five events I've attended in the past 2 months of July and August. Several observations that are playing with the mental health of all Veterans Groups everywhere in America and for that matter, anywhere Vietnam Veterans meet worldwide. Groups are facing a serious question. What happens as Vietnam Veterans continue our head-long fall, down the throat of mass genocide? This death march continues unabated and chapter after chapter of this group or post after post of that group, doesn't matter, all are fearful that The Vietnam Veteran population is plain and simple dying off, at an alarming rate. The living are asking a hard question, who will remember? What happens to the brand?

My chapter of VVA can't muster a Color Guard. VFWs are sharing meeting sites. This is causing a strange kind of fear.

No, not fear, but what I'm seeing in the eyes of both men and women is profound sadness. Our main and only support group, US VETS, is slipping through the wire and fading away with only a whimper of why. WHY us? This watching each other die-off is suffocating.

Our organizations can't make a month, 30 days until next meeting without announcing another Agent Orange (nerve gas-would have made Hitler proud) death. Agent Orange is chemical warfare waged by our government, industrial complex (corporations), military industrial complex and AMA against its own citizens. Two million have died horrible deaths. Families suffer and some die, and no records available. Blowing in the wind. Genocide of the warrior class.

The fear that anything about Vietnam, remembering anything about the war will simply just go away, and disappear without mention. Like almost no media coverage of Dec 7, 1941, Pearl Harbor Day, in 2019. Less is less is less, till, poof, there's left nothing, just silence. What war?

A major consideration for writing "Noble Canine", was TO CHRONICLE DAY TO DAY LIFE as a Sentry Dog Handler so that our jobs as handlers of the Noble German Shepherd in Vietnam is not lost to time. Through "Noble Canine", that records exists and chronicles training and night to night life of dog teams.

My busy July and August meetings I got to see a lot of Vietnam Veterans and their beautiful Brides. I have a special interest in the Wives, some are active in the VVA Auxiliary. I don't often sit through these meetings, a huge waste of time. I always end up feeling like I'm being scammed.

As our numbers grow fewer, the 'walking dead' are a lost generation.

Question: How does a whole army of Veterans just disappear! Is our silence, our acceptance, our permission?

Question: Will the few fighting to stay alive, the few remaining, will they roll over and just die, or will they stand?

Question: Is freedom worth the price of an "Agent Orange" death? NO, it is not!

What happens as most members die off, and chapter after chapter close their doors? A VFW Post Commander recently told me how his Post meets at another VFW Hall, due to fewer and fewer members.

In my twenty years of membership in Vietnam Dog Handlers Association, I've watched as our reunions were attended by few women. In time, that began to change and more women began to accompany their husbands to reunions. More and more of these wives, our brides, started attending more and more of our meetings. Today, at Vietnam Veteran reunions, it's mostly a veteran and his wife. Most Vietnam Veterans cannot function without some sort of assisting to her Veteran.

And men, listen up! We Veterans must reach out and embrace this concept of women leadership or all things Vietnam will...disappear!

Any group that represents military veterans is faced with its own extinction. Women see the future of her children and grandchildren, (left) in her hands and she must protect the future of the young.

I call on the current male leadership in ALL veteran groups to prepare the way for this change to take place and to allow it to flourish.

Some men will have a problem accepting a greater role for women's involvement in running the show. Better minds than this one, have been burning a lot of midnight computer time trying to figure out how to keep the doors open and the Vietnam Veteran commodity viable. Agent Orange is a bitch. Our Wives are the future. We men have no future!

Whether you agree or not, we are the 'walking dead' and a very loud clock is ticking, and the Twilight Zone is the home to our ghost. Men be nice and invite 'our better-halves' in to play and to lead. The time is upon us.

I just returned from a 2200 mile round-trip to Michigan and visited a fellow Sentry Dog Handler, BT, from a long time ago. My old friend and has aged gracefully. With the help of a cane, he gets around but on bad knees, but he gets around. Like all Vietnam Veterans, he is in a holy fight to stay alive. It's a daily battle. He's had other issues, some life threatening. We are both seventy-one years old, and live day to day. Barry enjoys his grandchildren and wants to be around when they are all growed-up.

At a VVA meeting and as I sit looking around at the VVA members enjoying tender-sweet BBQ, I noticed something in the eyes of the men and women in the room, fear! Not only do these men fear their own deaths from Agent Orange, but all of us have had to live with and watch, while thousands upon thousands of brothers experience premature deaths.

How much horror can a Vietnam Veteran endure? With 22 Veterans dying every day from suicide, I suggest, not much. Now, the only entities that offered any relief, like the DAV, VDHA, VVA, and others, don't have enough members to present a Color-Guard. These Clubs are dying, and the few surviving members are scared. The sadness I see in the room is in the eyes. What I see is chaos from so much suffering and dying. The hurt we feel, being betrayed by a lying (government), (military), (Veterans Administration), (medical community), (AMA) and, especially the American People. All are responsible for the deaths of two million Veterans. (FOREVER GENOCIDE)

Visiting the War Dog Memorial was the highlight of my week-long stay in Michigan.

Now, the only entities that offered any relief, like the DAV, VDHA, VVA, and others, don't have enough members to present a Color-Guard. (I know I'm repeating myself, but the message is too important to be taken lightly, let me be redundant on purpose).

As Vietnam Veterans die-off, so also will America die. I'm talking about the Spirit of America dies with ever Veteran's death. The old America will disappear and time will stop when the people of this country grow some balls and fight the chemical cartels and the oil cartels who are killing this planet. Global warming is a facade, is a huge cover-up to hide the real damage being done by these cartels. No difference between Agent Orange or GMO's, same poison, same chemistry, different day.

VA HOSPITAL, GAINESVILLE, FL

Joe

Monday May 21, 2012, (continued) 1:40 PM

Who's smarter, the Doctor, nurse, or patient? I wrote about the numbness earlier. I asked all involved and no one suggested this. Can being in one spot, even on this bed cause it? No one until Freddie said yes. I got him to pull sheet from my left side and cause me to roll to my right just a little. He did, and I immediately felt something different. I guess it was the blood flowing again. That is what caused the numbness. In 20 minutes, I was able to wiggle my toes. Another 10 minutes and I could move my whole leg a little more. I could move a little. I immediately started my bed exercises as prescribed my physical therapy dept.

It was improving at least until about 3 pm when my new bed arrived. It is the "Cadillac of all hospital beds" as described by manufacturer rep that was in my room. It probably is a great bed but everything needs a bit of adjustment or two. The CNA here is a wonderful lady named Paula. She was having a hard time raising the guard rail near my left shoulder. It would NOT stay up though she tried at least ten times. The factory rep stayed near the door looking disgusted with her complaining. He repeated several times, "It has to work. I lubed, adjusted and tried them all myself." CNA repeated, "I'm doing exactly what you are telling me and it won't stay." The factory rep guy finally came over to physically show her. First time he pulled it up it looked like it would stay, that is until he pulled on it and it fell.

He reset it again and left. Nurse Freddie came in unaware of this problem. He went to my left shoulder area to turn off nurse call button. He just touched that same guard rail and it fell. It scared me, Freddie and Paula. Freddie reset it and it seems to be staying.

May 23, 2012, 4 PM

The bed guy came. I guess he was trying to see if we wanted the old bed back. We should have. It was the same rude guy from yesterday. One of the nurses here noticed the mattress was about a foot lower in the bed frame then it should be. They used the overhead hoist system to raise me up, pull the mattress up, then lower me in the correct position. It felt a little better almost immediately. I started to exercise here in bed and got a little feeling back quickly. Not much, but a little. It was an improvement.

6:30 PM

This has to be my worst day ever. They decided to try to give me a shower. Both my legs are extremely swollen with very little feeling. They have to try to get me about 10 meters into the bathroom, washed, dried and back to bed. It's unbelievable. They are looking for a special harness to use on an overhead hoist system to get me there. Oh yea, I need a bowel movement too.

They got me to sit up on the side of the bed. The side rail was down on this new bed but sticks out a lot farther than on the older one, hurting my thighs very much. I tried to stand with the walker but could not. My legs were too numb and weak for me to stand at all. I almost fell on the floor. They tried to stop me from falling and had to grab me on both legs. The pain was unbelievable. They dragged me onto the bed yelling.

Finally, I could not breathe at all. I was writhing and fighting for a breath. They put me on 5 liters oxygen. I was still fighting. They tried to talk to me to calm down. There was no air at all going into my lungs. I was really panicking. They started to raise the head off the bed a little and the tiny breaths started to come. So slowly.

12 AM

It's hard to believe we just finished giving me a shower a little while ago. Had to use toilet too. I'm not sure I'll ever do either again the rest of my life. It took two male and one female nurse as well as an overhead electric lift system to accomplish all this. Oh yeah, two applications of 5 liters of oxygen too. They have special harnesses they need to get under me for the lift system. As they lift, it pulls on my body to lift, actually on the skin. Do you remember what Pemphigus affects? Yup, the skin. Hurts like hell, all over. As they raised and moved me, it pulled skin off in numerous locations, including most of my back, both sides at waist, left elbow and a few more I'll check on tomorrow. I'm not sure I'll ever try that again. I mean I can't come close to describing the pain. Something like being tortured by Taliban terrorists.

NOTHING IS HAPPENING!

Jimmie - Rant #11

1969, *Phu Cat AB Re-visited*

Truth be told, not until the first few days of January 1970 does the Kat finally get hit by enemy forces. But, surprise-surprise, for the first time NVA troops are lighting off ROCKETS while hiding in the mountains that surrounded Phu Cat. Got hit twice that night and you know from reading "Noble Canine, Search for the Edge", I slept through both attacks. I got out of Vietnam in the nick of time.

Fifty years ago this day I was a 'short-timer'. Eight months of being expendable as the first line of defense has probably taken a toll somehow, someway, that I am not aware of, yet. But going home, or better yet, leaving Vietnam is a reward all by itself. All my thoughts are of getting out of Vietnam in one piece, with all my body parts and all my mind intact. So far, so good. I, my comrades had no idea what was coming.

FYI, on this date fifty years ago, I was already infected by Agent Orange. Yes! I did leave Vietnam with the same me as I arrived with. What I had no understanding about, I left Vietnam whole in body, mind and spirit and carried a new hell back to the world. Entered through the gates of hell and started a journey as The Walking Dead. And for forty years I never knew Agent Orange was slowing having me for lunch from the inside out.

I was in total denial, that anything about Agent Orange had any validity. Not me, brother!

I came home from Vietnam, whole and ready to find my Bride and get on with life. All well, said and good, I stayed in a frozen state of raw ignorance for the next forty years. I loved life. But in 2009 the Dragon beast reared its ugly-fiery-breath, who flies at warp-speeds and IT entered my life, my home, my peace, and commenced to finish what the government and chemical cartel started, cleaning the slate of War Babies/Baby Boomers, but mostly...the 1%'$ had to destroy the victorious sons of WWII, war-baby-Warriors. Today, 2,000,000 dead baby-boomer-Warriors later? Nobody blinked. All baby boomers need to wake up and join the fight to save our planet from chemical poisoning. In fifty-years if we continue business as usual, it won't matter. It's always been about business and greed. The planet can't handle it anymore!

The Dragon never blinks, his mission of 'Gathering the Warrior Soul' is almost completed.

My refusal to learn all I could google about chemical warfare has cost me dearly. I flat refused to look the god-damned Beast in the eye, even aided and abetted, I did! But worse, my silence was my permission, a green light to start research on creating new earth foods. All this time, I was a card caring, life member of the Walking Dead. Now, this very day, A.O. equals G.M.O.'s. and our home planet is dying.

Had we understood the enemy, I am convinced, had I in the 1980's, while living in Hollywood, CA., and right in the middle of the Agent Orange court trails, with several hundred millions of dollars being stolen by slick lawyers, had I educated myself to all things Agent Orange, and also made the effort to educate others, more of the dead would be alive. More importantly the chemical cartel would not be in the food creating business of evil and death!

Dragon Brigade Forever

To any thinking Brigade member, do you realize in five years that most of our membership will be dead? Only a few thousand Dragon Brigade members will still be alive. We have a short time to act. The window of opportunity is open. Won't last?

So, why insult our Wives?

The President of Vietnam Veterans of America stated that Women will have NO LEADERSHIP ROLL IN VVA. In five years, our Women, our wives, will be the only humans around to pick-up the pieces and call to order the next VVA meeting. Why alienate our spouses. Only gatekeepers can answer. The fools! And you wonder where the men are? Lost.

Veteran groups must open their arms to these Women, the only souls left who care.

Why beat them up, they have suffered enough. Living with a Vietnam Veteran and chemical warfare victim is trial enough. For the most part, our women, our families, even generational family units have suffered. And By God, the world needs to hear about it. I insist! Dragon Brigade will have justice.

As always, share Noble Canine with your friends. It's OK to help this Vietnam Veteran, Agent Orange Victim, be successful. It's OK to help an Agent Orange Casualty and one of the Walking Dead who flat-out refuses to be a victim or lay down and just die. Dragon Brigade will have justice.

People who love Vietnam Veterans will not let Noble Canine melt away, and my desire to be #1 on the New York Times Best Sellers list is a fact waiting to happen. Noble Canine is an American Love story. Noble Canine is a U.S. Air Force Love story. Noble Canine expresses my Love of AnimalKind. Go, buy ten copies of the hardback and give them away at Christmas time.

VA HOSPITAL, GAINESVILLE, FL

Joe

May 24, 2012, 8:30 AM

Well, I guess I was really burned out from yesterday. A male nurse named Chris was here this morning and I guess I looked bad. I was sleeping, the breakfast tray was at my table and I was not moving. I was pretty out of it. He thought I was passed out again. This time when he tried to move me, it finally worked. I was pretty much out of it yesterday.

11:15 PM

A tech was just here. She's nice. She just told me last Monday my blood sugar grasped to 54. That's what made me pass out. Dr. told her because I was taking too much pain meds. I don't believe that. I was taking very little. I just told Jeff I want a morphine pump for pain. I must make it stop. I told Jeff and gave him full power of attorney because he may not like what I say, but I believe he will honor my decision, while I'm sure my brothers will not. They would do things out of love, what they think is best for me but not what I actually want. They don't know what 2 1/2 years of pain feels like.

May 28, 2012

It's about 5am and I'm awake again. Not sure if it's again or still awake, the pain is pretty bad. They ask us to give them a number to rate the pain from 1-10, as 10 being absolute worst. I just took a pretty strong pain pill about half hour ago but can't think of the name. I'm still at least a six, getting a little groggy but still at least a six. /AM I had breakfast about 7:30 today.

May 30, 2012, 3:30 AM

I think. I'm not real sure of the time. My skin seems much better, but at 180 mg of prednisone every day, I guess something has to happen. I've had a crappy day today. Nothing specific just feeling a real bad day. I think the prednisone and the mood swings has a lot to do with it. It's like big waves washing all over my body and I'm useless to stop it.

June 1, 2012

It's 1 AM what are YOU doing? You know I've mentioned several times in the past about my feelings including highly patriotic, those from my prednisone mood swings and as of 15 minutes ago, a sleeping pill I badly needed. I've had almost no sleep the past 4-5 nights causing near delusional episodes causing me serious concerns. If my sentences fall off somewhat or completely, that may be why. It's hard to concentrate right now.

It's about 6:30 PM now, still June 1. I guess I passed out awhile. In and out a few times, I guess. I was on the couch awhile too. Had dinner there. They just put me back in bed awhile. John (the RN) does a pretty good job getting me there and back alone.

I received a letter in the mail today from Willie in Oregon. It's great to hear from him and his wife. No cell phone. No email. No computer. It's like time stood still for him after invention of phone answering machine. In Oregon woods. Up on mountains. The best view of the USA imaginable. Having Elk, deer, moose, bear and caribou wander by while you sleep......it's like a dream.

It's about like the deer I shot a number of years ago in Mississippi with Billy Cheek. Boy I miss him. I was in a hunting stand he built overlooking a soybean field that was already harvested. It was a big field so I had a Remington 308 bolt action with 4X12X50 Simmons scope. Rather medium-priced scope but worked great for me. I also had a Sig Sauer 45ACP hand gun as it was my duty gun being a Deputy Sheriff.

First, three does came out to eat and looked rather relaxed. I could see the outline of another deer, unknown sex, in the bushes. After a few minutes it came out to eat the better food in the field. I could see it was a buck. The Remington was ready but I wanted to try the Sig 45. As he got closer, I eased the Remington into the corner as I drew the Sig. As I leveled the Sig on a broadside shot, the buck was about 30 feet away. One shot through the heart and he dropped like a rock. The bullet went 99.999% through, coming to a rest under bulging skin on the opposite side. I took one small slice with my hunting knife on the bulge and the mushroomed bullet dropped into my hand. Simply beautiful. I digress as Billy has since passed away from lung cancer.

BRIDES OF WARRIORS

Jimmie - Rant #12

2021

I had gone to the ballpark to walk. I can manage one trip around this half mile circle. Ladies' softball was in full swing and had most parking spaces taken. I finally pulled to a stop and just like that the sky opened and rain by the buckets ended women softball for the day.

But lately I've been enjoying all the rain, the storms, the winds, and lightning, all of it is pure magic. The air is energized, and the trees are happy. I know it's the result of pulling duty during monsoon season in Vietnam. I was already accustomed to heavy rains, from living in Florida, and I've survived hurricanes. I got married in a hurricane up in Pennsylvania in 1972. I love the rainy nights.

This rain was falling in long sheets, driven by fierce winds. People were running for shelter, which meant their cars for the most part. I was fascinated by the noise and rhythm, as large drops pounded the roof of the cab and I watched as strong winds moved rain about the parking lot at thirty to forty miles per hour. I hadn't seen such a downpour since Vietnam, and I couldn't see a thing and the truck shook from the windy conditions. I disappeared in the cab of my truck.

You reader, need to know, I started writing this blog entry three days ago. Five days now?! Not an easy subject for me!

Now, for the rest of the story.

I experienced a first ever flash-back, in that rainstorm and I was suddenly back at Phu Cat walking a dog in unimaginable rain, really, I was back walking post in Vietnam. As I set on my bucket, with torrential rains gushing everywhere, I became focused, and just like that, the rain stopped. On top of the clouds set a full-blown, full moon. That's when I saw me and Virginia in bed. In that flash of a second or two, it hit me hard the high price Agent Orange has suffered our marriage.

I'm also, back in my truck now, and not a soul is left in the ballpark, just me and the rain. The micro-flashback left me with a picture I will try and explain to you. I call it, 'love denied'! I took three days off, not writing, just thinking, but a lot of thinking!

This is what I come up with:

I can't hold my wife's hand without razor sharp spikes (fire ants) starting the process of pain release until my hand hurts so much that I have to pull away from her. Same for most parts of my body. I sleep with a pillow between my legs to keep shin bones from touching. This is ten years later. There has been no lovemaking. Agent Orange took that away also. Sometimes the pain from touching doesn't materialize for days or weeks at a time. You start feeling (sort-of) good for a change. But, as soon as I rollover and wrap my arm over her, invariably, I can feel the pain returning. I compare the nerve damage caused by Agent Orange to fire ants. Ten years later, I can bump a leg and just under the skin I can feel the heat rising, ever ready to eat flesh.

This is the life of a typical Vietnam Veteran, "the walking dead"!

I am so glad to be able to tell this story. It must be told and retold. A true story about betrayal. A country in denial. Citizens who turn their backs to a Holocaust right before their eyes. Why do you not see our deaths as more than a tragedy? The disgrace of America is deafening. Pathetic. True!

Do not forget Noble Brides, to be your warrior/Husbands' voices. Speak up, find your voice. Don't quit. Find your voice!

As I set in the truck, I was totally engulfed in a deluge of water and I begin to cry buckets as the realization hit me about my little 'tell-all' of 'love denied' to my wife. With two million dead warriors, most had wives. And all these wives have suffered and done without for so long, that they don't remember what lovemaking was like. When pain stands between you and the pleasures of touching, not lovemaking, just to be able to return the feelings of being able to hold your loved one. Agent Orange took that.

Agent Orange has reared its ugly head and a third generation is being infected with the disease. These are life-threatening events and it's all a big secret. My hope is these women, all Agent Orange survivors, join together and tell their stories until this country admits genocide. Until this country is so ashamed of the big-fake, the big-lie, so fed up with murder of the Warrior Class, this is no way for a government to treat its citizens. America must learn something from this genocide. It can happen to you, also. The 1%'$ eats the very flesh of its own, laughing all the way to the bank!

I'll close this rant by asking the 'Brides of Warriors' to write their stories. How lives are forever turned upside down as they are witnesses to the brutality and misery of another Agent Orange murder. If you do this and want to, please share your story with me, all I ask is a brief summation of the facts and I'll get back to you. Send to: Jimmie Moore, P.O. Box 55054, Jacksonville, FL. 32216.

VA HOSPITAL, GAINESVILLE, FL

Joe

June 2, 2012, 11:45 PM

I just can't shake it off, the sadness that is. The nurses and CNAs have been very good. The newest nurse tonight brought hot water so I could make instant coffee. Very nice of her. It is SO boring here it's unbelievable. If not for Internet and films, I'd go really crazy. I know it's very expensive due to Verizon "hotspot" coverages but I have no choice, really. The TV is too small and too far away.

The sadness continues like an onslaught of army ants with no end in sight. Is it the prednisone again or something else? I remember a while back I likened it to a wave washing across my body totally unstoppable. Maybe the sadness and boredom will pass. I hope so. Nurse is here now and I have to go. More later.

June 4, 2012

A new (new to me) student nurse named Vicky came in. Very nice. Small, pretty, big smile, actually quite beautiful, came in. We hit it off right away. I could feel her kindness right away. We talked a bit about her, her husband, future plans, etc. I was intrigued about her plans for a clinic in South America, for helping the poor with health concerns and spreading the word of God whenever possible.

June 6, 2012, 8:45 PM

I think it was last Sunday the 3rd of June, for unknown reasons my sugar crashed again. I don't know the number but it was a really big problem. What I recall is when I did wake-up, I was "totally blind." I could see nothing at all. I was scared. I could hear people talking and running all around me. I was told that a nurse had to feed me, I'm assuming food or juice or sugar packs. I don't recall. After a while I was starting to see outlines and a few colors but not much else. White then yellow and some bright orange became visible. Where was I? What was happening? I was asking these questions over and over but I was not sure who I was asking or who was there. I got no response. Little by little my vision was clearing, but oh so slowly. First the outlines, then a few facial features. Finally, I could tell if it was male or female and who it was. What I don't know yet is how long all this took. Was it minutes or hours? How near death was I? Did anyone call Jeff? I WILL find out.

10:00 PM

I just spoke with Jeff and no one called him from this hospital at all. I'll talk with the nurse here in a few minutes and see how bad I really was and put that here. Like I said earlier and they have in my records here, Jeff has a full P.O.A on me and the last word on what happens to me.

10:10 PM

Sorry but still waiting for the nurse. They are pretty busy here. I'll be up until about 12 AM. More later.

I just found out my sugar was 80. That's a bit low for you but pretty low for me. Regular patients are at risk below 70. They put me at risk below 100. It was bad but just above critical for me. If it was critical, I'd have been stabilized then moved to another floor. I was not moved. I'm still in 311E. One of the doctors here, maybe Dr. Rush, told me there was a problem with my meds. He changed some and reduced others. I know he reduced my prednisone as well as the insulin. I remember he once told me I was taking 90 units of insulin in one form or another. He told me that on Friday.

June 9, 2012. Saturday 09:45 AM

I just finished having breakfast. Dr. Do was just here. He said I'm scheduled to leave here Monday morning. A Nursing home

I think right across the street from this place wants me if I have Medicaid, I think. Of course, this place will help me apply for what I need.

I was feeling OK today. It seems I'm more of an evening or afternoon person. I just feel so-so when I wake up but much better towards afternoon or evening, actually drawing energy from those around me in the evening until I finally crash myself.

It seems these drugs, especially prednisone, are causing huge changes in my blood sugar from 589 highs to 40's lows. Everyone in this hospital is on warning if their sugar drops to 70. They have mine set at 100 as warning number level. Once it passes that number it's difficult to stop it. I'm feeling sleepy right now. I was up all night. Just couldn't sleep.

Joseph Barbarise no longer wrote in his Journal and passed away in June, 2012.

OUR CHILDREN, WHO STANDS FOR THEM?

Jimmie - Rant #13

2021

You're truly blessed, I said to a veteran on Facebook. Me, likewise blessed. Most Veterans are denied due process of Justice. I have a retired Navy man-neighbor, who lost over 60% use of his lungs. Why? Working, overhauling ships, the VA denied him his rights to justice, fair pay and benefits. This is rampant, pandemic in the Veteran Community. Because I cannot work, I have a 100% rating. I'll tell all you Veterans something, this small chicken-shit pension the VA bestowed on me does not buy my silence. It's not even a down-payment. If you have buried friends because Agent Orange took their lives to damn early, especially if you are receiving financial assistance from the VA, then stand. For Truth, Justice, and the American Way. Two million Vietnam Veterans are dead, and still the pain and the suffering of chemical warfare is lived behind closed doors, closed lives. I'm tired of being the 'wiped boy', the 'scapegoat', for a lying government, lying medical cartel, lying VA and that goes double for lying military. Who, dear Veteran, will stand with our wives and children? When there are not enough Vietnam Veterans for a decent color guard? Who stands for the left-behind? Don't you know, dear Veteran? Agent Orange is found in 2nd, 3rd generations of our children. Who in hell's name will stand for our progeny?

From a long time ago.

I did not want to see the Sixties end. I loved the music scene and played the drums in a successful high school party band. The country was abuzz with change. Freedom marchers, and freedom fighters, women's rights, voters' rights, civil rights, Cuban Crises, race to the moon and end the war and bring the troops home. And lest we forget, assassinations. All done by Baby Boomers. By the time I got to Vietnam, I was probably more hippy than airman. More hippies were serving in all branches and dying in Vietnam. The draft had much to do with hippies in uniform.

I still say the greatest ambassadors America has ever produced continue to be the men and women of our armed forces. Wherever our troops are stationed in the world, there goes the soul/spirit of America.

It takes seven support personnel to put one fighting man in the front lines engaging the enemy. That's what I heard. The rest of us were support and few saw actual combat in Vietnam. So, the rich American kids (to the Vietnamese all G.I.'s where rich 19-year old's) propped-up the economy of South Vietnam. Most Americans even in wartime are generous. Vietnam was flooded with nineteen-year-old strangers, singing rock and roll. I was one of those 'young men', I even purchased a pair of drum sticks at the BX and took them with me at night, while on duty.

But, as a Sentry Dog Handler, my life and my psyche and the lives of sixty-two dog teams were tested, every night.

The handler climbed down from the deuce-and-a-half, and gently lifted his German Shepherd to the ground. He sits, locked-and-loaded his weapon (Car-15), finished the dogs change-over, from choke chain to leather working collar, for Junior (Smokey-X480) and as I removed his muzzle, I set on my bucket and watched the last flicker of taillights disappear down the runway berm-road. This 10,000-foot-long runway required a lot of dog team power.

As I remain seated, I considered what lay in my path tonight as I entered the zone (Kilo-anything) I radioed with base-command and checked-in that Kilo-43 was secured. I would have no more contact with Base unless Junior alerted. I was on my own, all alone and scared but the night and this patch of holy ground, belonged to me. Here I was, a 'tin-god', I carried a full-automatic baby M-16 in my left hand, and a Sentry Dog leashed to my right wrist and for the next ten hours we played hide-and-seek. "Where the hell is Charlie?"

At Phu Cat Air Base our F-4 Phantoms supported Marines and Grunts all the way to the DMZ. The enemy's goal was to blow our bomb and fuel-dumps, located on the northeast side of the base. Destroy even one or the other, and our aircraft are out of action, and it takes time to re-supply, which means no aircraft overhead supporting Americans on the ground from Phu Cat. Cobra Flight was the other 'mad-dog' working the night, but Team "Noble Canine" was first line of defense. "Where others feared to tread, Canine walked alone!" Thanks, Vernon, for that quote!

I worked 360 nights at the Cat, leashed to a fearless, indispensable, highly intelligent, supremely trained Sentry Dog. In all I spent 360 nights leashed to this powerful killing machine. I even learned to talk dog, and to listen. 3600 hours of bonding with these Noble Canine. Training and working these dogs were the 'high-life' for me, I wouldn't trade the experience for anything. I learned to love all AnimalKind because of these Noble German Shepherd. What a dog!

With the end of my one-year tour of duty, 1969 came to an end. And I left Vietnam on January 05, 1970 for the world, and the sixties came to an end, and with it a special event was finished. Complete. 'Goodnight Mr. American Pie'?

Jimmie Moore
Author, Light-worker and Imaginator
Noble Canine, Search for the Edge.

PEACE DUKE II, PEACE!

Jimmie Rant - #14

1969 Phu Cat Revisited

Fifty years ago at Phu Cat Air Base February 22, 1969 From a blog post at moorek9.com

Number one, the Blog page I did on Joe Barbarise needed time to settle. And I needed some input on the post I created.

Number two, I had made my peace with Duke II.

Number three, Feb. 22, 1969, Phu Cat AB was hit by a ground force of VC sappers.

I expect push-back on the AO expose' of the pain and suffering that huge numbers of Vietnam Veterans have endured due to Agent Orange poisoning. But mostly, this nation has been shielded from the truth. The truth is too big for weak minds. Worst, we Veterans who suffer, silently, seem to take some strange and perverse satisfaction at enduring male-stoic passivity. I don't get it. I'm mad as hell and, why the hell aren't veterans up in arms. How many friends, buddies, comrades in arms, what-ever you call a Vietnam Veteran, how many brothers must we watch being reduced to the walking dead.

I wonder when Veterans Groups start raising money for yet another memorial, latest memorial to Agent Orange victims. 'Oh boy! A whole new agenda. Gee-golly, we can build memorials all over America. That will keep the membership focused for a while.' While Veterans organizations pretend doing good for all Veterans, except the sick ones. I'm here to tell you our numbers are less than 400,000 and the 'walking dead' is dying off right before your eyes.

Oh! Duke II, you poor dumb dog.

You would have made a hell of a pet for a family with kids and a big fenced-in yard. Ever since that night SSgt. Frances ran a practice alert by coming on my post and seeing at what point Duke would alert, well, Duke II never alerted and sealed his fate that night.

Before Sergeant Frances mounted up to leave, I asked, "What was going to happen to Duke, will they send him somewhere he can receive more training?" Yeah?! I'm naïve.

Frances just looked for a long second, grinned, slammed the jeep into gear, "Moore, what will most likely happen to your dog is he will be sent to Saigon and put down."

"That's it?!" I asked.

Frances drove off, and I was left looking down at Duke, thinking about my dog being put down. Oh! shit boy. If this is the Air Force way of dealing with a sub-standard Sentry Dog, whom am I to complain. I've risked my life for six weeks, it's time to get a real MWD and put Duke II out to pasture.

It took a little time to sink in, and when I realized Duke's nights were numbered, I could no longer be mad at the animal. In fact, I accepted that Duke II would never harm another, to protect me or any other handler, and it would cost him his life.

BUT, a part of me didn't care.

That night, February 22, 1969, we got hit. Duke's fate was sealed. I would load Duke II for the plane ride south to Tan Son Nhut AB which was located right in the middle of the capital city of South Vietnam, Saigon.

But the longest night of my life lay right here in front of me, right now.

Early shift had departed their usual time and a group of us were just returning from supper. The alarm went out, the base is under attack, you've ten minutes to get ready for work and be at the pick-up point. Move it, move it!

Intruders are inside the wire, one handler down.

FINAL RANT ABOUT JOSEPH LOUIS BARBARISE

Jimmie - Rant #15

2021

Did I tell you that my friend Joe grew up in Secaucus, New Jersey? There are a lot of Barbarise's in northern Jersey. I visited with Vinny the last few days of our thirty-day leave. I was stationed in New Jersey, Vinny headed west to Travis AFB a little east of Napa, CA. Vince is a retired local Law Enforcement and both his sons followed in his footsteps. Joe headed to Florida and Eglin AFB and made Florida his home. He was a medically retired Sheriff's Deputy and made his home in Orlando. Joe loved and respected womenkind. He learned to love animalkind in Vietnam. And as an animal photographer, he excelled, putting his life at risk on several occasions with big cats and a bull to get the pictures.

I spent some time with Joe, visiting almost weekly for the nine months he lived. Joe was the second Agent Orange death I had comforted. Both were horrible deaths. Neither Vietnam Veteran received compensation from Veterans Administration. Joe was trying to get Social Security monies the whole time he was in VA hospitals. A few weeks before his death he received a letter from Social Security informing him that he would have to travel to Orlando S.S. office to complete the paperwork. Joe would have to travel by ambulance and still naked as a j-bird, just to satisfy some useless bureaucrat. Why couldn't the Social Security Administration send a representative a mere hundred miles north to Gainesville or the hundred miles to Tampa or better yet, when Joe was shipped to Orlando, where was Social Security Administration? At the Veterans Administration no one was talking about benefits.

I've often wondered how many Vietnam Veterans suffered the way Joe suffered. For the staff at Tampa VA, I don't think this was the first time seeing a body so ravished by chemical warfare as Joe was, they took it in stride. I watched intertly the stage performance and the lead roll Joe was playing. When Joe was finally relieved of his filthy traveling cloths and set naked, everyone had the same reaction I did. Just could not believe the horror I saw.

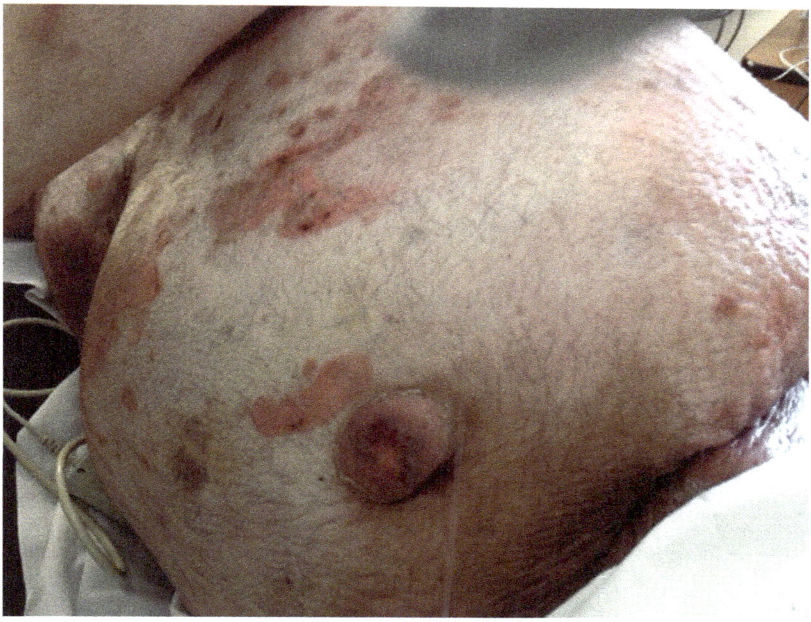

Joe was black and blue with lose skin hanging from different parts of his body, raw oozing sores covered his back and the back of his legs. All his limbs where grossly swollen. His elbow had a softball size blister that would open and ooze soon enough. His face was covered with dead skin and open sores. On top of this he topped the scales at 300 pounds. Joe never wore clothing again, not even underwear to cover his nakedness To work with

Joe required physical strength on the staff's part. A lift was used to move Joe to and from the bathroom. Part of his treatment plan was a daily shower, with special soaps to wash the hair and the skin. Joe was in constant pain and heavily medicated. Joe was also bored out of his mind. His new smartphone was a life saver letting him watch movies to kill a lot of empty time. But movies being streamed via his Apple iPhone was expensive. From day one, back in America, Joe sought out assistance from the VA and SSA. Both failed him. Is there no shame at the Veterans Administration? None! The medical community on every level, has failed the American People. The medical whores are responsible for two million dead Airmen, Sailors, Soldiers, Marines and Coastie's. The USA has become unhealthy, sick, and dying. As citizens, we must demand healing, not more pills from pharmakia, the chemistry of evil, all based on oil.

He Ain't Heavy, He's my Brother!

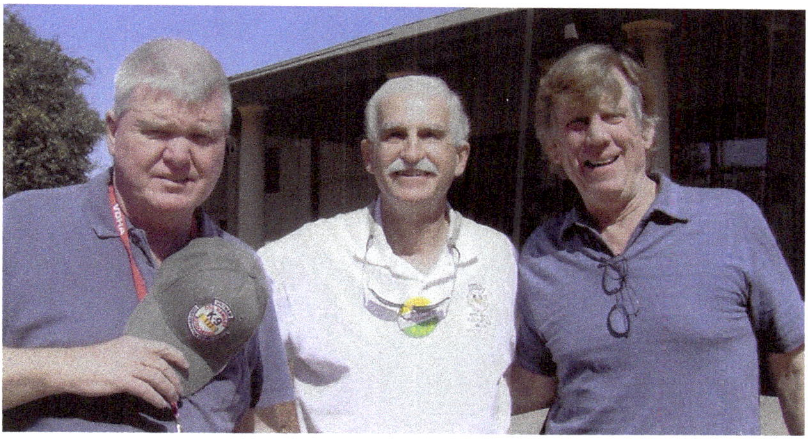

50 Years Friends

John, Vince and myself are at Lackland Air Force Base in San Antonia, TX. Another reunion. We look pretty good for the older set. We still have our hair, which was a big deal to us airmen chasing after WAF during our Sentry Dog School days, way back in 68. We are in pretty good health. 2009 the Dragon landed at my home and hasn't left yet. Vince and John have never had problems with Agent Orange. Vince was my best man in 1972, and that's when he told about his daughter having skin problems. Joe will never attend a reunion with us.

More at:

moorek9.com
moorek9.com/blog

CPSIA information can be obtained
at www.ICGtesting.com
Printed in the USA
LVHW081242131121
702999LV00036B/774

9 781732 671935